ARCO
PROFESSIONAL CAREER EXAMINATION SERIES

Second Edition

NURSING
COMPREHENSIVE
EXAMINATION REVIEW

BY GEORGE HOREMIS, M.D. & CLEMENCIA MATAMORS, R.N.

Arco Publishing Company, Inc.

New York

Second Edition, Second Printing, 1977

Published by Arco Publishing Company, Inc.
219 Park Avenue South, New York, N.Y. 10003

Library of Congress Cataloging in Publication Data

Horemis, George.
  Nursing comprehensive exam review.

  Includes bibliographical references.
  1. Nursing—Examinations, questions, etc.
I. Matamors, Clemencia, joint author. II. Title.
[DNLM: 1. Nursing—Examination questions.
WY18 H811n]
RT55.H67 1976   610.73′076   76-14822
ISBN 0-668-02499-2 pbk.

Printed in the United States of America

Contents

Introduction

This completely revised and updated edition of *Nursing Comprehensive Examination Review* provides new material in each subject chapter plus two additional chapters entitled Psychiatry (Chapter Six) and History and Law (Chapter Ten).

It consists of multiple-choice questions with referenced answers which provide excellent study material. Each subject is covered in a separate chapter. The references provided will help students and graduates to review any of the subjects.

Variations of the standard multiple-choice question form are included in order to familiarize the reader with the most common types of questions found on actual examinations. The nurse who wishes to make the best use of this book should not be satisfied with merely determining the correct answer to a given question but should also do additional research on the alternate choices for the same questions. In this way, she will broaden her background while at the same time, strengthen her knowledge in areas in which she may be deficient.

Adequate preparation for an examination also requires a thorough review of the subjects from standard textbooks. This book is intended not to replace these textbooks, but to supplement them.*

*For in-depth examination review, the following books are also available from Arco:
Child Health Nursing Review by Luz S. Porter, R.N., Ph.D.
Maternal Health Nursing Review by Josephine Sagebeer, R.N., C.N.M., M.S.
Psychiatric/Mental Health Nursing Review by Janet A. Rodgers, R.N., Ph.D., and Weslee N. McGovern, R.N., M.A.
Nutrition and Diet Therapy Nursing Review by Lorraine S. Boykin, Ed.D., R.N.
Medical-Surgical Nursing Review by Mary E. Hazzard, B.S.N., Ph.D.

References

On the last line of each test item, at the right hand side, there appears a number combination that identifies the reference source and the page(s) where information pertaining to the question and answer may be found. The first number refers to the reference source, the second to the pages. For example: (1:135) is a reference to page 135 in the first text on the list, Chaffee's *Basic Physiology and Anatomy*.

1. Chaffee, Ellen E.; Greisheimer, Esther M. *Basic Physiology and Anatomy,* second edition, J.B. Lippincott Co., Philadelphia: 1969.
2. Smith, Alice Lorraine. *Principles of Microbiology,* sixth edition, The C.V. Mosby Co., St. Louis: 1969.
3. Bergersen, Betty S.; Goth, Andres. *Pharmacology in Nursing,* twelfth edition, The C.V. Mosby Co., St. Louis: 1973.
4. Diamond, Sheldon R. *Fundamental Concepts of Modern Physics,* first edition, Amsco School Publications, Inc., New York: 1970.
5. John, Lewis R. *College Chemistry,* ninth edition, Barnes and Noble Books, New York: 1971.
6. Fitzpatrick, Elise; et al. *Maternity Nursing,* twelfth edition, J.B. Lippincott Co., Philadelphia: 1971.
7. Broadribb, Violet. *Foundations of Pediatric Nursing,* second edition, J.B. Lippincott Co., Philadelphia: 1973.
8. Krause, Marie V.; Hunscher, Martha A. *Food, Nutrition and Diet Therapy,* eighth edition, W.B. Saunders Co., Philadelphia: 1972.
9. Schafer, Kathleen Neuton; et al. *Medical-Surgical Nursing,* fifth edition, The C.V. Mosby Co., St. Louis: 1971.
10. Griffin, Gerald Joseph; Griffin, Joanne King. *History and Trends of Professional Nursing,* seventh edition, The C.V. Mosby Co., St Louis: 1973.
11. Creighton, Helen. *Law Every Nurse Should Know,* second edition, W.B. Saunders Co., Philadelphia: 1970.
12. Matheney, Ruth V.; Topalis, Mary. *Psychiatric Nursing,* fifth edition, The C.V. Mosby Co., St. Louis: 1970.
13. Freeman, Ruth B. *Community Health Nursing Practice,* W.B. Saunders Co., Philadelphia: 1970.

Chapter One

Anatomy and Physiology

Directions: Select from among the lettered choices the ONE that most appropriately answers the question or completes the statement.

1. All of the following are found in the temporal bone *except* the

   A. styloid process
   B. alveolar process
   C. zygoma
   D. mastoid process
   E. auditory meatus   (1:69)

2. The haversian canals are associated with

   A. elastic cartilage
   B. fibrous cartilage
   C. smooth muscle
   D. bone
   E. none of the above   (1:65)

3. The body is divided into upper and lower portions by a

   A. coronal plane
   B. sagittal plane
   C. lateral plane
   D. transverse plane
   E. frontal plane   (1:7)

4. All the following are parts of the temporal bone *except* the

   A. mastoid process
   B. auditory meatus
   C. xiphoid process
   D. styloid process
   E. zygoma   (1:70, 71)

5. How many carpal bones are there in the upper extremity?

   A. 4
   B. 5
   C. 6
   D. 7
   E. 8   (1:94)

6. The acetabulum is associated with the head of the

   A. humerus
   B. tibia
   C. femur
   D. fibula
   E. ulna   (1:96)

7. What is the normal number of paired ribs?

   A. 7
   B. 8
   C. 9
   D. 12
   E. 14   (1:86)

8. The mental foramen of the mandible transmits the

   A. trochlear nerve
   B. palatine nerve
   C. abducens nerve
   D. optic nerve
   E. none of the above   (1:76)

9. The patella is also called the

   A. kneecap
   B. talus

C. tarsus
D. ischium
E. atlas   (1:95)

10. The longest bone of the body is the

    A. tibia
    B. fibula
    C. spine
    D. ulna
    E. femur   (1:97)

11. The talus is a bone in the

    A. head
    B. thigh
    C. foot
    D. back
    E. chest   (1:102)

12. The clavicle is also called the

    A. frontal bone
    B. scapula
    C. collar bone
    D. occipital bone
    E. scaphoid bone   (1:88)

13. How many fontanels are normally present
    at birth?

    A. 3
    B. 4
    C. 5
    D. 6
    E. 8   (1:79)

14. The ulna is a bone in the

    A. forearm
    B. upper arm
    C. leg
    D. thigh
    E. neck   (1:92)

15. The fibula is a bone in the

    A. hand
    B. foot
    C. leg
    D. back
    E. thorax   (1:102)

16. Approximately how many bones are found
    in the human skeleton?

    A. 100
    B. 200
    C. 150
    D. 250
    E. 75   (1:68)

17. Which of the following muscles arise from
    the coracoid process?

    A. brachialis
    B. triceps brachii
    C. sartorius
    D. biceps brevis
    E. palmaris longus   (1:152)

18. The buccinator muscle is associated with
    the

    A. neck
    B. scalp
    C. mouth
    D. thorax
    E. forearm   (1:173)

19. The hamstring muscles include

    A. the biceps fermoris
    B. the semitendinosis
    C. the semimembranosis
    D. all of the above
    E. none of the above   (1:165)

20. The procerus muscle is found in the

    A. mouth
    B. neck
    C. hand
    D. nose
    E. thigh   (1:172)

21. The piriformis muscle is associated with
    the

    A. thorax
    B. neck
    C. nose
    D. ear
    E. thigh   (1:183)

22. All of the following are muscles of the nose
    except the

A. procerus
B. corrugator
C. depressor septi
D. nasalis
E. dilatator naris anterior   (1:172)

23. The pelvic floor is called the

A. procerus
B. perineum
C. peritoneum
D. myometrium
E. none of the above   (1:161)

24. Sugar is found in the blood in the form of

A. sucrose
B. galactose
C. glucose
D. cellulose
E. maltose   (1:308)

25. The first heart sound is caused by the

A. opening of the aortic valve
B. opening of the pulmonary valve
C. closing of the A-V valves
D. vibration of the ventricles
E. all of the above   (1:337)

26. The blood volume in the adult is approximately

A. 2000 ml
B. 3000 ml
C. 4000 ml
D. 5000 ml
E. none of the above   (1:297)

27. The average life span of the red blood cells is

A. 120 days
B. 50 days
C. 15 days
D. 8 days
E. 24 hours   (1:303)

28. Stagnant hypoxia can be caused by any of the following except

A. cyanide poisoning
B. shock

C. cardiac failure
D. arterial embolism
E. rupture of the heart   (1:441)

29. The clinical picture observed in carbon monoxide poisoning is due to

A. hemolysis
B. hypokalemia
C. a chemical union of the carbon monoxide with the hemoglobin of the red cells
D. transformation of the carbon monoxide to carbon dioxide in the blood
E. arrest of oxidation in the tissues by enzyme interference   (1:301)

30. Which of the following substances inhibits the production of prothrombin in the liver?

A. heparin
B. Dicoumarol ®
C. vitamin K
D. vitamin C
E. glucose   (1:312)

31. Monocytes constitute what percentage of the total number of white cells?

A. 2%
B. 3%
C. 3% to 8%
D. 10%
E. 15% to 20%   (1:304)

32. About what percentage of plasma is protein?

A. 3%
B. 5%
C. 6% to 8%
D. 9%
E. 10% to 12%   (1:306)

33. What is the approximate diameter of the red blood cells?

A. 2 microns
B. 4 microns
C. 6 to 9 microns
D. 10 to 12 microns
E. 25 microns   (1:301)

34. Normal bleeding time is approximately

    A. 1 to 4 min.
    B. 5 to 7 min.
    C. 8 to 10 min.
    D. 10 to 12 min.
    E. 12 to 15 min.   (1:310)

35. What is the approximate percentage of water found in blood plasma?

    A. 65
    B. 72
    C. 80
    D. 85
    E. 92   (1:307)

36. The normal coagulation time of the blood is

    A. 30 to 40 sec.
    B. 40 to 60 sec.
    C. 1 to 2 min.
    D. 3 to 10 min.
    E. 15 to 20 min.   (1:310)

37. Semilunar valves are found in the

    A. coronary sinus
    B. inferior vena cava
    C. superior vena cava
    D. aorta
    E. subclavian artery   (1:325)

38. How many cusps does the mitral valve have?

    A. 2
    B. 3
    C. 4
    D. 5
    E. 6   (1:324)

39. The lingual artery is a branch of the

    A. superior thyroid artery
    B. external carotid artery
    C. internal carotid artery
    D. facial artery
    E. none of the above   (1:354)

40. The internal mammary artery arises from the

    A. subclavian artery
    B. axillary artery
    C. innominate artery
    D. vertebral artery
    E. thyroid artery   (1:356)

41. The thoracic duct empties into the

    A. superior vena cava
    B. inferior vena cava
    C. left subclavian vein
    D. aorta
    E. azygos vein   (1:381)

42. The internal jugular vein is a continuation of the

    A. carotid sinus
    B. cavernous sinus
    C. sinus venosus
    D. sigmoid sinus
    E. petrosal sinus   (1:368)

43. The following can be said about the bronchial arteries

    A. they originate from the aorta
    B. they are branches of the pulmonary arteries
    C. they originate from the subclavian arteries
    D. they are branches of the vertebral arteries
    E. there are four bronchial arteries in each lung   (1:358)

44. Branches of the external carotid include which of the following arteries?

    A. the lingual
    B. the facial
    C. the occipital
    D. the maxillary
    E. all of the above   (1:353, 354)

45. The respiratory rate in the adult is usually

    A. 8/min.
    B. 10/min.
    C. 12 to 14/min.
    D. 14 to 18/min.
    E. 18 to 22/min.   (1:436)

46. The average tidal volume is

    A. 4000 ml
    B. 3000 ml
    C.   500 ml
    D.   200 ml
    E. 1500 ml   (1:436)

47. The percentage of carbon dioxide in the expired air is

    A. 4.40%
    B. 2%
    C. 0.04%
    D. 16%
    E. 21%   (1:440)

48. The volume of air that moves in and out of the lungs with each respiratory movement is called

    A. vital capacity
    B. expiratory reserve
    C. inspiratory reserve
    D. tidal volume
    E. residual air   (1:436)

49. The largest of the following pulmonary volumes is the

    A. tidal volume
    B. residual volume
    C. vital capacity
    D. inspiratory reserve
    E. expiratory reserve   (1:436)

50. The inspiratory reserve volume is about

    A.   200 ml
    B.   300 ml
    C. 1000 ml
    D. 3000 ml
    E. 6000 ml   (1:436)

51. The normal atmospheric pressure is

    A. 600 mm Hg
    B. 760 mm Hg
    C. 780 mm Hg
    D. 560 mm Hg
    E. 582 mm Hg   (1:428)

52. The smallest of the following pulmonary volumes is the

    A. residual volume
    B. tidal volume
    C. vital capacity
    D. inspiratory reserve volume
    E. expiratory reserve volume (1:436,440)

53. Most of the carbon dioxide in the blood is carried as

    A. carbonic acid in the plasma
    B. carbon dioxide in the plasma
    C. carbonate ions
    D. bicarbonate ions
    E. none of the above   (1:441)

54. The vital capacity of the average adult is about

    A. 6000 ml
    B. 4500 ml
    C. 3000 ml
    D. 2000 ml
    E. 1500 ml   (1:436)

55. The residual volume of air in the lungs of an adult is about

    A.   150 ml
    B.   500 ml
    C. 1000 ml
    D. 3000 ml
    E. 1500 ml   (1:440)

56. How much oxygen can be combined with one gram of hemoglobin?

    A. 13.4 ml
    B. 134 ml
    C. 1340 ml
    D. 0.13 ml
    E. 1.34 ml   (1:441)

57. The largest cartilage of the larynx is the

    A. arytenoid
    B. cricoid
    C. thyroid
    D. epiglottic
    E. none of the above   (1:420)

58. Hiccup is a spasmodic contraction of the

    A. intercostal muscles
    B. rectus muscles
    C. muscles of the larynx
    D. diaphragm
    E. none of the above   (1:433)

59. The organ called the throat is the

    A. trachea
    B. pharynx
    C. larynx
    D. tonsil
    E. epiglottis   (1:419)

60. How many cartilages make up the larynx?

    A. 2
    B. 3
    C. 6
    D. 9
    E. 14   (1:420)

61. The laryngeal prominence known as the "Adam's apple" is the

    A. thyroid cartilage
    B. epiglottis
    C. cricoid cartilage
    D. cuneiform cartilage
    E. trachea   (1:422)

62. The nerves of the larynx are derived from the

    A. trigeminal nerve
    B. vagus nerve
    C. facial nerve
    D. obturator nerve
    E. phrenic   (1:422)

63. All of the following structures are found in the mediastinum except the

    A. thoracic aorta
    B. heart
    C. thymus
    D. pulmonary veins
    E. bronchi   (1:425)

64. The adenoids are located in the

    A. nasopharynx
    B. oropharynx
    C. nasal vestibule
    D. oral vestibule
    E. vomer   (1:419)

65. All the following are paranasal sinuses except the

    A. frontal
    B. maxillary
    C. ethmoidal
    D. sagittal
    E. sphenoidal   (1:418)

66. The space between the lungs is called

    A. pericardium
    B. peritoneum
    C. mediastinum
    D. sternum
    E. vomer   (1:425)

67. Temporary cessation of breathing is called

    A. asthma
    B. anoxia
    C. eupnea
    D. dyspnea
    E. apnea   (1:431)

68. A gram of protein is equivalent to

    A. 12 calories
    B.   8 calories
    C.   6 calories
    D.   4 calories
    E.   2 calories   (1:502)

69. An enzyme which acts upon fats is called a

    A. lipase
    B. protease
    C. pepsin
    D. phosphatase
    E. gastrin   (1:490)

70. The parietal cells of the stomach secrete

    A. mucin
    B. pepsin
    C. lipase
    D. hydrochloric acid
    E. trypsin   (1:469)

71. The crypts of Lieberkühn are found at the

    A. intestines
    B. gall bladder
    C. mouth
    D. trachea
    E. vagina (1:470)

72. Kupffer's cells are found in the

    A. ovaries
    B. liver
    C. kidneys
    D. eye
    E. adrenal glands (1:478)

73. Brunner's glands are found in the

    A. cecum
    B. pharynx
    C. duodenum
    D. sigmoid colon
    E. ear (1:470)

74. Approximately how many pounds does the liver weigh in the adult?

    A. 2 lbs
    B. 3 lbs
    C. 4.5 lbs
    D. 6 lbs
    E. 7 lbs (1:470)

75. The gall bladder

    A. has a capacity of 40 to 50 ml
    B. is pear-shaped
    C. stores and concentrates bile
    D. all of the above
    E. none of the above (1:479)

76. The duct of Wirsung is found at the

    A. liver
    B. spleen
    C. pancreas
    D. sigmoid colon
    E. ileum (1:481)

77. Approximately how long is the small intestine?

    A. 3 ft

    B. 7 ft
    C. 12 ft
    D. 23 ft
    E. 33 ft (1:469)

78. Peyer's patches are found in the

    A. peritoneum
    B. pleura
    C. small intestine
    D. liver
    E. large intestine (1:470)

79. Glisson's capsule is found in the

    A. spleen
    B. kidney
    C. pancreas
    D. duodenum
    E. liver (1:474)

80. What is the approximate length of the esophagus in inches?

    A. 4
    B. 6
    C. 7
    D. 10
    E. 13 (1:466)

81. The phrenic nerve receives fibers from the

    A. third cervical spinal nerve
    B. fourth cervical spinal nerve
    C. fifth cervical spinal nerve
    D. all of the above
    E. none of the above (1:209)

82. Wharton's duct is associated with the

    A. pancreas
    B. duodenum
    C. submandibular salivary gland
    D. sublingual salivary gland
    E. parotid gland (1:466)

83. How many pairs of salivary glands are there?

    A. 2
    B. 3
    C. 4
    D. 5
    E. 8 (1:466)

84. Which of the following promotes reabsorption of sodium chloride in the kidneys?

    A. epinephrine
    B. parathormone
    C. aldosterone
    D. cortisone
    E. glucagon   (1:599)

85. Approximately how many nephrons does the normal kidney have?

    A.   100,000
    B.   200,000
    C.   500,000
    D. 1,000,000
    E. 5,000,000   (1:526)

86. The entire muscular coat of the urinary bladder is called the

    A. serratus muscle
    B. detrusor muscle
    C. procerus muscle
    D. trigone of the bladder
    E. longus colli muscle   (1:530)

87. The loop of Henle is found in the

    A. stomach
    B. kidney
    C. thyroid gland
    D. inner ear
    E. external ear   (1:526)

88. Intraocular pressure is normally

    A.   5 mm Hg
    B. 10 mm Hg
    C. 12 to 14 mm Hg
    D. 15 mm Hg
    E. 20 to 25 mm Hg   (1:278)

89. The brain stem includes

    A. the medulla
    B. the pons
    C. the midbrain
    D. all of the above
    E. none of the above   (1:222)

90. There are how many pairs of spinal nerves?

    A. 24
    B. 26
    C. 28
    D. 31
    E. 33   (1:207)

91. The bone or bones which form the walls of the orbit includes

    A. the palatine bone
    B. the sphenoid bone
    C. the ethmoid bone
    D. all of the above
    E. none of the above   (1:288)

92. The membranous labyrinth contains

    A. the cochlear duct
    B. the utricle
    C. the saccule
    D. all of the above
    E. none of the above   (1:288)

93. The average volume of the cerebrospinal fluid in man is

    A.   10 ml
    B.   25 ml
    C.   55 ml
    D. 100 ml
    E. 135 ml   (1:236)

94. Parkinsonism is associated with

    A. tremor
    B. diffuse rigidity
    C. lesions of the basal ganglia
    D. all of the above
    E. none of the above   (1:234)

95. The respiratory center lies at the

    A. cerebellum
    B. cerebral cortex
    C. medulla
    D. pons
    E. midbrain   (1:240)

96. The smallest cranial nerve is the

    A. optic nerve
    B. olfactory nerve

C. trochlear nerve
D. vagus nerve
E. facial nerve   (1:240)

97. The eighth cranial nerve is called the

A. optic nerve
B. auditory nerve
C. vagus nerve
D. olfactory nerve
E. hypoglossal nerve   (1:242)

98. Nerve deafness may be the result of injury to the

A. olfactory nerve
B. vagus nerve
C. trochlear nerve
D. spinal cord
E. auditory nerve   (1:291)

99. The stapes is

A. a bone of the neck
B. a bone of the ear
C. a bone of the foot
D. an endocrine gland
E. none of the above   (1:288)

100. Strabismus is

A. the colored part of the eye
B. the middle coat of the eye
C. a deviation of one of the eyes due to a muscle defect
D. the white part of the eye
E. none of the above   (1:280)

101. The receptors for hearing are located in the

A. auditory canal
B. auricle
C. inner ear
D. ear drum
E. eustachian tube   (1:287)

102. Testosterone is secreted by the

A. prostate
B. pituitary gland
C. kidney
D. adrenal medulla
E. testes   (1:572)

103. Lack of iodine in the diet may cause

A. simple goiter
B. scurvy
C. pellagra
D. anemia
E. tetany   (1:556)

104. Which of the following stimulates contractions of the uterine muscle?

A. oxytocin
B. insulin
C. testosterone
D. somatotrophin
E. none of the above   (1:552)

105. Increased pigmentation of the skin can be caused by hyperfunction of the

A. adrenal mebulla
B. thymus
C. adrenal cortex
D. thyroid
E. pancreas   (1:561)

106. Insulin

A. is a hormone
B. lowers the blood sugar
C. makes glucose available for glycogen formation in the liver
D. is produced in the pancreas
E. all of the above   (1:562,564)

107. The glucose tolerance test detects disturbances in

A. kidney function
B. pancreatic function
C. gall bladder function
D. uterine function
E. heart function   (1:563)

108. Heat is lost from the body principally by

A. radiation
B. perspiration
C. conduction
D. convection
E. cutaneous vasoconstriction   (1:512)

109. The following organs belong to the female reproductive system except the

    A. ovaries
    B. vagina
    C. vulva
    D. mammary glands
    E. uterus   (1:577)

110. The spermatic cord contains

    A. the testicular arteries
    B. the ductus deferens
    C. veins
    D. nerves
    E. all of the above   (1:575)

111. The mammary gland has how many lobes?

    A. 3
    B. 6
    C. 8 to 10
    D. 15 to 20
    E. 25 to 30   (1:589)

112. The portion of the uterus above the entrance of the uterine tubes is called

    A. fornix
    B. fundus
    C. vestibule
    D. Cowper's fold
    E. pudental cleft   (1:581)

113. What structure produces spermatozoa?

    A. prostate
    B. seminiferous tubules
    C. spermatic cord
    D. ductus deferens
    E. epididymis   (1:570)

114. Fertilization usually occurs in the

    A. cervix of the uterus
    B. vagina
    C. fundus of the uterus
    D. ovary
    E. fallopian tube   (1:591)

115. The uterus

    A. is a hollow organ

    B. is pear-shaped
    C. is located in the pelvic cavity
    D. all of the above
    E. none of the above   (1:580)

116. The Douglas fold is found at the

    A. pericardium
    B. palmar fascia
    C. rete testis
    D. recto-uterine area
    E. inguinal canal   (1:581)

117. Most cases of obesity in adults are due to

    A. thyroid deficiency
    B. pituitary deficiency
    C. overeating in terms of total caloric intake
    D. excess protein ingestion
    E. pancreatic insufficiency   (1:504)

118. The BSP (bromsulphalein) test is used to determine

    A. liver function
    B. cardiac function
    C. the pH of the blood
    D. kidney function
    E. genital function   (1:481)

Answer the questions in this group by following the directions below. Select

    A. **if only A is correct**
    B. **if only B is correct**
    C. **if both A and B are correct**
    D. **If neither A nor B is correct**

119. The atlas
    A. is the first cervical vertebra
    B. articulates with the occipital bone
    C. both
    D. neither   (1:81)

120. Mast cells

    A. are connective tissue cells
    B. contain histamine
    C. both
    D. neither   (1:43)

121. Hyaline cartilage

    A. is pearly white
    B. is the most common type of cartilage
    C. both
    D. neither   (1:44,45)

122. Cartilage

    A. contains chondrocytes
    B. has a rich blood supply
    C. both
    D. neither   (1:44)

123. The atlas

    A. is the first cervical vertebra
    B. has no body
    C. both
    D. neither   (1:81)

124. The radius is

    A. a bone of the leg
    B. longer than the femur
    C. both
    D. neither   (1:93)

125. The thoracic vertebrae

    A. are twelve in number
    B. articulate with the ribs
    C. both
    D. neither   (1:83)

126. The lumbar vertebrae have

    A. short spinous processes
    B. transverse foramina
    C. both
    D. neither   (1:83)

127. The spine

    A. encloses the spinal cord
    B. is composed of 23 bones
    C. both
    D. neither   (1:80,81)

128. The female pelvis is generally

    A. wider than the male pelvis
    B. lighter than the male pelvis
    C. both
    D. neither   (1:95)

129. Paired bones of the cranium include the

    A. ethmoid
    B. parietal
    C. both
    D. neither   (1:69)

130. The triceps brachii is the antagonist of the

    A. biceps
    B. brachialis
    C. both
    D. neither   (1:152)

131. The genioglossus muscle

    A. arises from the hyoid bone
    B. forms part of the body of the tongue
    C. both
    D. neither   (1:144)

132 Muscles inserted in the radius include the

    A. trapezius
    B. serratus anterior
    C. both
    D. neither   (1:148,150)

133. Muscles inserted in the ulna include the

    A. triceps brachii
    B. pronator teres
    C. both
    D. neither   (1:152,254)

134. Muscles inserted in the radius include the

    A. supinator
    B. teres minor
    C. both
    D. neither   (1:177)

135. The quadratus femoris muscle

    A. originates from the ischial tuberosity
    B. rotates the thigh medially
    C. both
    D. neither   (1:183)

136. Muscles flexing the leg include

    A. the popliteus
    B. the gastrocnemius
    C. both
    D. neither   (1:185)

137. The gammaglobulins of the plasma

    A. are produced by the basophil cells
    B. are important in providing immunity against certain diseases
    C. both
    D. neither   (1:307)

138. Fibrinogen

    A. is a plasma protein
    B. is essential to the clotting mechanism of the blood
    C. both
    D. neither   (1:309)

139. Granular leukocytes originate from

    A. the bone marrow
    B. the lymph nodes
    C. both
    D. neither   (1:305)

140. The lymphocytes are formed in

    A. the lymph nodes
    B. the bone marrow
    C. both
    D. neither   (1:305)

141. Granular leukocytes include

    A. lymphocytes
    B. monocytes
    C. both
    D. neither   (1:304,305)

142. A normal differential white blood count shows

    A. 65% neutrophiles
    B. 26% lymphocytes
    C. both
    D. neither   (1:303)

143. Normal plasma contains

    A. glucose

    B. uric acid
    C. both
    D. neither   (1:310)

144. Branches of the external carotid artery include

    A. the internal maxillary artery
    B. the anterior cerebral artery
    C. both
    D. neither   (1:354)

145. Branches of the internal carotid artery include

    A. the pharyngeal artery
    B. the middle cerebral artery
    C. both
    D. neither   (1:354)

146. The superior mesenteric artery

    A. arises from the internal iliac artery
    B. supplies the descending colon
    C. both
    D. neither   (1:358,362)

147. Parietal branches of the abdominal aorta include

    A. the inferior phrenic arteries
    B. the lumbar arteries
    C. both
    D. neither   (1:362)

148. The thoracic duct

    A. begins at the level of the second lumbar vertebra
    B. receives lymph from all parts of the body below the diaphragm
    C. both
    D. neither   (1:381)

149. The lymphocytes

    A. are formed in the lymphoid tissues
    B. have a life span of 15 hours
    C. both
    D. neither   (1:305,306)

150. Hemoglobin contains

   A. cobalt
   B. iron
   C. both
   D. neither   (1:301)

151. Bilirubin and biliverdin are derived from

   A. the white blood cells
   B. the platelets
   C. both
   D. neither   (1:480)

152. The second heart sound

   A. occurs at the end of the systole
   B. is caused by the closing of the aortic and pulmonary valves
   C. both
   D. neither   (1:337)

153. Normal plasma contains

   A. glucose
   B. uric acid
   C. both
   D. neither   (1:310,311)

154. Fibrinogen

   A. is a plasma protein
   B. is essential to the clotting mechanism of the blood
   C. both
   D. neither   (1:307)

155. The cardiac output

   A. is about 5 liters/min at rest
   B. decreases in case of anemia
   C. both
   D. neither   (1:332)

156. The deep veins of the lower limbs are

   A. the long saphenous vein
   B. the short saphenous vein
   C. both
   D. neither   (1:371)

157. The deep veins of the lower limbs

   A. follow the corresponding major arteries
   B. have no valves
   C. both
   D. neither   (1:371)

158. The coronary arteries arise from

   A. the ascending aorta
   B. the arch of the aorta
   C. both
   D. neither   (1:329)

159. The femoral artery

   A. supplies the muscles of the thigh
   B. is a continuation of the internal iliac artery
   C. both
   D. neither   (1:362)

160. The pulmonary veins

   A. empty into the left atrium
   B. contain oxygenated blood
   C. both
   D. neither   (1:348)

161. Hemorrhage causes

   A. acceleration of the heart rate
   B. hypertension
   C. both
   D. neither   (1:410)

162. The dorsalis pedis artery

   A. is a continuation of the anterior tibial artery
   B. has no branches in the foot
   C. both
   D. neither   (1:362)

163. Heart murmurs

   A. are soft sounds
   B. may be due to stenosis of a cardiac valve
   C. both
   D. neither   (1:337)

164. The blood is

   A. dark red in the arteries
   B. bright red in the veins

C. both
D. neither   (1:297)

165. A repolarization wave of the ECG is represented by

    A. the P wave
    B. the T wave
    C. both
    D. neither   (1:335)

166. The sino-atrial node is

    A. the "pacemaker" of the heart
    B. located in the right atrium
    C. both
    D. neither   (1:326)

167. Red blood cells

    A. are formed in the bone marrow
    B. carry oxygen and carbon dioxide
    C. both
    D. neither   (1:301)

168. During inspiration

    A. the lungs expand
    B. the antero-posterior diameter of the thorax decreases
    C. both
    D. neither   (1:429)

169. In pneumothorax

    A. the intrapleural pressure becomes equal to that of the atmosphere
    B. the lung collapses
    C. both
    D. neither   (1:433)

170. "Barrel chest" is associated with

    A. pulmonary emphysema
    B. pregnancy
    C. both
    D. neither   (1:428)

171. Openings in the walls of the nasopharynx include

    A. the two posterior nares
    B. the two auditory tubes
    C. both
    D. neither   (1:419)

172. The palatine tonsils

    A. are masses of lymphatic tissue
    B. are located in the nasopharynx
    C. both
    D. neither   (1:419)

173. Pneumothorax

    A. refers to the presence of air in the pleura
    B. may occur spontaneously as a result of lung disease
    C. both
    D. neither   (1:433)

174. The epiglottis

    A. closes the opening into the larynx during the act of swallowing
    B. is a leaf-shaped cartilage
    C. both
    D. neither   (1:420)

175. The trachea

    A. is two inches long
    B. commences at the lower border of the cricoid cartilage
    C. both
    D. neither   (1:423,424)

176. Ptyalin

    A. initiates the digestion of starch
    B. acts on protein
    C. both
    D. neither   (1:484)

177. The liver

    A. stores sugar as glycogen
    B. secretes bile
    C. both
    D. neither   (1:480)

178. Parts of the stomach include

    A. the fundus

B. the pylorus
C. both
D. neither   (1:467)

179. The permanent teeth

A. appear between 4 and 6 years
B. number 32
C. both
D. neither   (1:464)

180. The large intestine

A. is about 5 ft long
B. has a sacculated appearance
C. both
D. neither   (1:471)

181. Bile salts

A. are formed from cholesterol
B. help in the absorption of fatty acids
C. both
D. neither   (1:480)

182. Bile is important for the digestion of

A. sugars
B. protein
C. both
D. neither   (1:480)

183. The liver

A. is the largest organ of the body
B. is located in the left hypochondriac region
C. both
D. neither   (1:474)

184. The liver

A. has 6 lobes
B. maintains homeostasis of glucose in the blood
C. both
D. neither   (1:480)

185. Saliva

A. protects the mouth against drying
B. commences the digestion of fat

C. both
D. neither   (1:484)

186. The pancreas is

A. an exocrine gland
B. an endocrine gland
C. both
D. neither   (1:481)

187. The pancreas

A. is located in the epigastric and left hypochondriac regions of the abdomen
B. is composed of lobules
C. both
D. neither   (1:481)

188. The small intestine

A. is 10 ft. long
B. is attached to the stomach by cartilage
C. both
D. neither   (1:469)

189. The large intestine in the adult

A. has a diameter of 2½ inches
B. is longer than the small intestine
C. both
D. neither   (1:471)

190. The Taeniae coli are found in

A. the rectum
B. the appendix
C. both
D. neither   (1:472)

191. The rectum

A. is about 5 cm long
B. extends from the sigmoid colon to the anal canal
C. both
D. neither   (1:472)

192. Abnormal constituents of urine include

A. blood
B. ketone bodies
C. both
D. neither   (1:537)

193. Normal urine contains

    A. sugar
    B. bile
    C. both
    D. neither   (1:537)

194. Organic constituents of the normal urine include

    A. urea
    B. creatinine
    C. both
    D. neither   (1:95)

195. The ureters

    A. connect the kidneys with the bladder
    B. are located behind the parietal peritoneum
    C. both
    D. neither   (1:529)

196. The urinary bladder

    A. serves as a reservoir for urine until it is to be discharged
    B. has two openings
    C. both
    D. neither   (1:530)

197. The kidneys

    A. have a bean-shaped appearance
    B. are located in the anterior part of the abdominal cavity
    C. both
    D. neither   (1:522)

198. The renal medulla

    A. is the inner portion of the kidney
    B. contains the capsule of Bowman
    C. both
    D. neither   (1:522)

199. The female urethra

    A. is 6 inches long
    B. lies immediately in front of the vagina
    C. both
    D. neither   (1:532)

200. Miotic drugs include

    A. homatropine
    B. pilocarpine
    C. both
    D. neither   (1:284,285)

201. The cornea

    A. is the colored part of the eye
    B. has no blood vessels
    C. both
    D. neither   (1:272)

202. Abnormalities of the cerebellum may result in

    A. loss of coordination
    B. loss of equilibrium
    C. both
    D. neither   (1:223)

203. If the vagi nerves are cut

    A. the heart rate decreases
    B. the force of contraction of the heart decreases
    C. both
    D. neither   (1:329)

204. Sympathetic stimulation causes

    A. dilation of the coronary arteries
    B. acceleration of the heart
    C. both
    D. neither   (1:255)

205. Drugs that constrict the pupil of the eye include

    A. cocaine
    B. epinephrine
    C. both
    D. neither   (1:284)

206. The sciatic nerve

    A. is the longest nerve in the body
    B. is the main branch of the sacral plexus
    C. both
    D. neither   (1:213)

207. The common peroneal nerve supplies

    A. the lateral muscles of the leg
    B. the dorsal muscles of the foot
    C. both
    D. neither   (1:213)

208. The medulla oblongata

    A. is a conduction pathway
    B. lies between the pons and the mid-brain
    C. both
    D. neither   (1:222)

209. Branches of the trigeminal nerve include

    A. the ophthalmic nerve
    B. the maxillary nerve
    C. both
    D. neither   (1:240)

210. Openings found in the fourth ventricle of the brain include

    A. the foramina of Luschka
    B. the foramen of Magendie
    C. both
    D. neither   (1:238)

211. The third ventricle of the brain

    A. is located between the medulla and the pons
    B. communicates with the lateral ventricle through the foramen of Monroe
    C. both
    D. neither   (1:238)

212. The aqueous humor

    A. is drained into the blood through the canal of Schlemm
    B. fills the space behind the lens
    C. both
    D. neither   (1:278)

213. The vitreous body

    A. fills the space between the cornea and the iris

    B. helps to maintain the shape of the eyeball
    C. both
    D. neither   (1:278)

214. In the spinal cord

    A. the white matter is located centrally
    B. the white matter is composed of neuron cell bodies
    C. both
    D. neither   (1:207)

215. Ascending pathways of the spinal cord include

    A. the dorsal spinocerebellar tract
    B. the ventral spinothalamic tract
    C. both
    D. neither   (1:216)

216. Injury to the hypoglossal nerve causes

    A. difficulty in speaking
    B. difficulty in swallowing
    C. both
    D. neither   (1:242)

217. Descending tracts of the spinal cord include

    A. the dorsal spinocerebellar tract
    B. the pyramidal tract
    C. both
    D. neither   (1:216)

218. The lacrimal gland

    A. is the size and shape of an almond
    B. drains into the upper portion of the nasal cavity
    C. both
    D. neither   (1:273)

219. The iris

    A. is located between the cornea and the lens
    B. contains 3 sheets of smooth muscle
    C. both
    D. neither   (1:274)

220. The middle ear

    A. communicates with the mastoid air cells
    B. is an air cavity in the temporal bone
    C. both
    D. neither   (1:287)

Each statement is followed by four suggested answers. Answer according to the following key:

    A. if answers 1, 2, and 3 are correct
    B. if 1 and 3 are correct
    C. if 2 and 4 are correct
    D. if only 4 is correct
    E. if all are correct

221. Transitional epithelium

    1. is the most abundant of all the primary tissues
    2. forms the lining of the urinary bladder
    3. forms the lining of the respiratory tract
    4. is found in structures which are subject to periodic distention   (1:41)

222. The dermis is

    1. also called corium
    2. also called true skin
    3. composed of connective tissue
    4. the surface layer of the skin   (1:48)

223. Sebaceous cutaneous glands are found in the

    1. neck
    2. palms
    3. axilla
    4. soles   (1:50)

224. Sweat glands

    1. are found over the entire skin
    2. are located in the dermis
    3. are more numerous in the palms and soles
    4. number about 5 million in the skin of an adult   (1:50)

225. Certain connective tissue cells

    1. store fat
    2. ingest bacteria
    3. produce antibodies
    4. produce heparin   (1:42)

226. Goblet cells secrete

    1. heparin
    2. DNA
    3. myosin
    4. mucous   (1:38)

227. The skin performs many functions such as

    1. protection of underlying tissues
    2. temperature regulation
    3. excretion of waste products
    4. vitamin D formation   (1:52)

228. Long bones

    1. are found in the extremities
    2. have a shaft or diaphysis
    3. have a medullary cavity
    4. have two epiphyses   (1:59)

229. Short bones are located in the

    1. neck
    2. wrist
    3. leg
    4. ankle   (1:59)

230. Air sinus(es) *not* communicating with the nasal cavity is/are the

    1. maxillary
    2. sphenoid
    3. frontal
    4. mastoid   (1:70)

231. Air sinuses communicating with the nasal cavity include the

    1. ethmoid
    2. sphenoid
    3. frontal
    4. mastoid   (1:75)

232. The ligamenta flava connects the lamina of the

    1. cervical vertebrae
    2. thoracic vertebrae

3. lumbar vertebrae
4. coccyx   (1:86)

233. In the adult, hipbone is formed by the fusion of

1. ilium
2. ischium
3. os pubis
4. sacrum   (1:94)

234. Muscles associated with the nose include the

1. zygomatic
2. orbicularis oris
3. frontalis
4. dilatores naris   (1:141)

235. Superficial veins of the lower extremity include the

1. great saphenous vein
2. popliteal vein
3. small saphenous vein
4. posterior tibial veins   (1:370,371)

236. Deep veins of the lower extremity include the

1. posterior tibial veins
2. anterior tibial veins
3. popliteal vein
4. femoral vein   (1:370,372)

237. Deep veins of the upper extremity include the

1. radial veins
2. brachial veins
3. axillary vein
4. cephalic vein   (1:368,369)

238. Superficial veins of the upper extremity include the

1. ulnar vein
2. basilic vein
3. subclavian vein
4. cephalic   (1:368,369,370)

239. Unpaired cranial venous sinuses include the

1. superior sagittal
2. transverse
3. occipital
4. superior sagittal   (1:366)

240. Paired cranial venous sinuses include the

1. inferior sagittal
2. inferior petrosal
3. straight
4. cavernous   (1:366,368)

241. Branches of the internal carotid artery include the

1. ophthalmic artery
2. posterior communicating artery
3. anterior cerebral artery
4. middle cerebral artery   (1:354)

242. Major branches of the subclavian artery include the

1. vertebral artery
2. internal mammary artery
3. thyrocervical trunk
4. anterior cerebral artery   (1:356,357)

243. The walls of arteries include the

1. tunica intima
2. tunica media
3. tunica adventitia (external)
4. tunica parietal   (1:344)

244. Layers of the heart wall include the

1. endocardium
2. myocardium
3. epicardium
4. omentum   (1:323)

245. The right atrium of the heart

1. is larger than the left atrium
2. has thinner walls than the left atrium
3. receives blood from the upper portion of the body via the superior vena cava
4. does not receive blood from the lower portion of the body   (1:324)

246. The left atrium of the heart

    1. has thicker walls than the right atrium
    2. receives blood from the lungs
    3. communicates to the left ventricle through the mitral valve
    4. receives blood from the lower part of the body   (1:324)

247. The inferior vena cava receives blood from the following veins

    1. common iliac
    2. spermatic
    3. renal
    4. hepatic   (1:373,374)

248. The portal system of veins drain blood from the

    1. spleen
    2. stomach
    3. pancreas
    4. gallbladder   (1:374)

249. Branches of the celiac artery include the

    1. hepatic artery
    2. left gastric artery
    3. splenic artery
    4. superior phrenic arteries   (1:358)

250. The superior mesenteric artery supplies the

    1. duodenum
    2. jejunum
    3. sigmoid
    4. cecum   (1:360)

251. The inferior mesenteric artery supplies the

    1. left half of the transverse colon
    2. descending colon
    3. sigmoid colon
    4. most of the rectum   (1:362)

252. Parietal branches of the abdominal aorta include the

    1. inferior phrenic arteries
    2. lumbar arteries
    3. middle sacral artery
    4. spermatic arteries   (:362)

253. Branches of the thoracic aorta include the

    1. pericardial arteries
    2. bronchial arteries
    3. esophageal arteries
    4. intercostal arteries   (1:358)

254. Branches of the abdominal aorta include the

    1. renal arteries
    2. ovarian arteries
    3. suprarenal arteries
    4. superior mesenteric artery   (1:358)

255. Branches of the ascending aorta include the

    1. right coronary artery
    2. right subclavian artery
    3. left coronary artery
    4. vertebral arteries   (1:352)

256. Branches of the aortic arch include the

    1. left common carotid artery
    2. left subclavian artery
    3. innominate artery
    4. pericardial arteries   (1:352)

257. The external ear

    1. is 1½ inches long
    2. extends from the auricle to the tympanic membrane
    3. has ceruminous glands
    4. communicates with the pharynx by way of the auditory tube   (1:287)

258. The tympanic membrane

    1. is covered by skin
    2. is also called ear drum
    3. can vibrate with sound waves
    4. contains the receptors for position sense   (1:287)

259. The middle ear contains

    1. air
    2. the malleus
    3. the incus
    4. the staples   (1:287,288)

260. The bony labyrinth includes the

    1. cochlea
    2. vestibule
    3. semicircular canals
    4. mastoid air cells   (1:287,288)

261. The pigment that determines the color of the eye is found in the

    1. pupil
    2. lens
    3. anterior chamber
    4. iris   (1:27)

262. The nervous part of the retina is made up of

    1. ganglion cells
    2. bipolar cells
    3. cones and rods
    4. epithelial cells   (1:275)

263. The corpuscles of Meissner are concerned with

    1. pressure
    2. heat
    3. cold
    4. touch   (1:264)

264. The corpuscles of Ruffini are concerned with

    1. touch
    2. pressure
    3. cold
    4. heat   (1:265)

265. Receptors for pressure are the corpuscles of

    1. Meissner
    2. Krause
    3. Ruffini
    4. Vater-Pacini   (1:264)

266. Sympathetic stimulation causes

    1. enlargement of the pupil
    2. contraction of the radial muscle of the iris
    3. increased activity of sweat glands
    4. increased intestinal peristalsis (1:255)

267. In the spinal cord the

    1. gray matter is located centrally
    2. gray matter is composed of cell bodies
    3. gray matter contains unmyelinated nerve fibers
    4. white matter surrounds the gray matter   (1:207)

268. Example(s) of motor cranial nerves is/are the

    1. oculomotor nerve
    2. trochlear nerve
    3. hypoglossal nerve
    4. vagus verve   (1:240,243)

269. The trigeminal nerve innervates the

    1. teeth
    2. mucous membranes in the head
    3. skin in the head
    4. intercostal muscles   (1:246)

270. The facial nerve branches out in the

    1. muscles of the face
    2. submaxillary glands
    3. sublingual glands
    4. taste buds of the tongue   (1:247)

271. The vagus nerve branches out in the

    1. larynx
    2. pharynx
    3. coronary arteries
    4. pancreas   (1:247)

272. The vagus nerve

    1. is the tenth cranial nerve
    2. contains motor fibers
    3. contains sensory fibers
    4. contains somatic and visceral fibers   (1:243)

273. Examples of sensory cranial nerves include the

    1. auditory nerve
    2. vagus nerve
    3. optic nerve
    4. hypoglossal nerve   (1:242,243)

274. Openings of the fourth ventricle of the brain include the

   1. foramina of Lushka
   2. foramen of Monroe
   3. foramen of Magendie
   4. foramen ovale   (1:238)

275. Signs of oculomotor nerve damage are

   1. drooping (ptosis) of the upper eyelid
   2. dilation of the pupil
   3. turning of the eyeball downward and outward
   4. ptosis of the corner of the mouth   (1:240)

276. The subarachnoid fluid fills the

   1. ventricles of the brain
   2. subarachnoid spaces around the brain
   3. subarachnoid spaces around the spinal cord
   4. middle ear   (1:236)

277. The subarachnoid fluid contains

   1. potassium
   2. a large amount of protein
   3. sodium
   4. a large number of red blood cells   (1:236)

278. Sensory portions of the trigeminal nerve include the

   1. maxillary nerve
   2. mandibular nerve
   3. ophthalmic nerve
   4. optic nerve   (1:240)

279. Which of the following belong to the basal ganglia?

   1. caudate nucleus
   2. lentiform nucleus
   3. putamen
   4. globus pallidus   (1:228)

280. The glossopharyngeal nerves

   1. arise from the spinal cord
   2. arise from the medulla oblongata
   3. supply the muscles of the neck
   4. branch out in the tongue and the pharynx   (1:242)

Directions: Each group of numbered words and statements is followed by the same number of lettered words, phrases or statements. For each numbered word or statement choose the lettered item that is most closely related to it.

Questions 281 to 285
281. Rectus abdominis
282. Gluteus medius
283. Pectoralis major
284. Masseter
285. Psoas major

   A. It extends from the sternum to the pubis
   B. It is inserted into the mandible
   C. It is inserted into the greater trochanter
   D. It is inserted into the humerus
   E. It is inserted into the smaller trochanter of the humerus   (1:174,181,183)

Questions 286 to 290
286. Deltoid muscle
287. Gluteus maximus muscle
288. Pectoralis major muscle
289. Sternocleidomastoid muscle
290. Risorius muscle

   A. It retracts the angle of the mouth outward
   B. Flexes head when both muscles act together on the chest
   C. It extends the femur
   D. It adducts the humerus
   E. It abducts the upper arm   (1:174,176,177,183)

Questions 291 to 295
291. Olfactory nerve
292. Optic nerve
293. Trigeminal nerve
294. Facial nerve
295. Vagus nerve

   A. Tenth cranial nerve
   B. Fifth cranial nerve
   C. Second cranial nerve

D. First cranial nerve
E. Seventh cranial nerve (1:240,242,243)

Questions 296 to 300

296. Oculomotor nerve
297. Hypoglossal nerve
298. Glossopharyngeal nerve
299. Statoacoustic nerve
300. Abducens nerve

A. Third cranial nerve
B. Ninth cranial nerve
C. Sixth cranial nerve
D. Eighth cranial nerve
E. Twelfth cranial nerve (1:240,242,243)

Answer Key: Anatomy and Physiology

1. B	39. B	77. D	115. D	153. C	191. B	229. C	267. E
2. D	40. A	78. C	116. D	154. C	192. C	230. D	268. A
3. D	41. C	79. E	117. C	155. A	193. D	231. A	269. A
4. C	42. D	80. D	118. A	156. D	194. C	232. A	270. E
5. E	43. A	81. E	119. C	157. A	195. C	233. A	271. E
6. C	44. E	82. C	120. C	158. A	196. A	234. D	272. E
7. D	45. D	83. B	121. C	159. C	197. A	235. B	273. B
8. E	46. C	84. C	122. A	160. C	198. A	236. E	274. B
9. A	47. A	85. D	123. C	161. A	199. B	237. A	275. A
10. E	48. D	86. B	124. D	162. A	200. B	238. C	276. A
11. C	49. C	87. B	125. C	163. C	201. B	239. B	277. B
12. C	50. D	88. E	126. A	164. D	202. C	240. B	278. B
13. D	51. B	89. D	127. A	165. A	203. B	241. E	279. E
14. A	52. B	90. D	128. C	166. C	204. A	242. A	280. C
15. C	53. D	91. D	129. B	167. C	205. D	243. A	281. A
16. B	54. B	92. D	130. C	168. A	206. C	244. A	282. C
17. D	55. E	93. E	131. B	169. C	207. C	245. A	283. D
18. C	56. E	94. D	132. D	170. A	208. A	246. A	284. B
19. D	57. C	95. C	133. C	171. C	209. C	247. E	285. E
20. D	58. D	96. C	134. A	172. A	210. C	248. E	286. E
21. E	59. B	97. B	135. A	173. C	211. B	249. A	287. C
22. B	60. D	98. E	136. C	174. C	212. A	250. C	288. D
23. B	61. A	99. B	137. B	175. B	213. B	251. E	289. B
24. C	62. B	100. C	138. C	176. A	214. D	252. A	290. A
25. E	63. E	101. C	139. A	177. C	215. C	253. A	291. D
26. D	64. A	102. E	140. A	178. C	216. C	254. E	292. C
27. A	65. D	103. A	141. D	179. B	217. B	255. B	293. B
28. A	66. C	104. A	142. C	180. C	218. A	256. A	294. E
29. C	67. E	105. C	143. C	181. C	219. A	257. A	295. A
30. B	68. D	106. D	144. A	182. D	220. C	258. A	296. A
31. C	69. A	107. B	145. B	183. A	221. C	259. E	297. E
32. C	70. D	108. A	146. D	184. B	222. A	260. A	298. B
33. C	71. A	109. D	147. C	185. A	223. B	261. D	299. D
34. A	72. B	110. E	148. C	186. C	224. A	262. A	300. C
35. E	73. C	111. D	149. C	187. C	225. E	263. D	
36. D	74. B	112. B	150. B	188. D	226. D	264. D	
37. D	75. D	113. B	151. D	189. A	227. E	265. D	
38. A	76. C	114. E	152. C	190. D	228. E	266. E	

Chapter Two

Microbiology

Directions: Select from among the lettered choices the one that most appropriately answers the question or completes the statement.

1. Outbreaks of sore throat due to contaminated milk are caused by organisms of the genus

   A. Streptococcus
   B. Brucella
   C. Staphylococcus
   D. Treponema
   E. Salmonella   (2:570)

2. Malta fever is a synonym for

   A. diphtheria
   B. scarlet fever
   C. brucellosis
   D. cholera
   E. yellow fever   (2:363)

3. Loeffler's medium is generally used for the isolation of

   A. *E. coli*
   B. *C. diphtheriae*
   C. *B. abortus*
   D. *S. viridans*
   E. *H. influenzae*   (2:328)

4. Petragnani's medium is generally used for the cultivation of

   A. *M. tuberculosis*
   B. *N. gonorrheae*
   C. *H. pertussis*
   D. *S. bovis*
   E. *E. coli*   (2:104)

5. The fertile hen's egg is generally used as a culture medium for

   A. spirochetes
   B. pneumococci
   C. viruses
   D. anaerobes
   E. neisseriae   (2:430)

6. Tellurite medium is used for the isolation of

   A. *C. diphtheriae*
   B. *B. abortus*
   C. *E. coli*
   D. *S. lactis*
   E. *N. gonorrheae*   (2:322)

7. The Weil-Felix test is valuable in the diagnosis of

   A. malaria
   B. typhoid fever
   C. whooping cough
   D. tetanus
   E. none of the above   (2:187)

8. The Frei test is used to diagnose

   A. pulmonary tuberculosis
   B. syphilis
   C. lymphogranuloma venereum
   D. gonorrhea
   E. trichinosis   (2:469)

9. The Neufeld reaction is generally used in the typing of

   A. viruses
   B. streptococci

27

C. pneumococci
D. Salmonella
E. staphylococci   (2:308)

10. The small bodies present in the microorganisms producing diphtheria are called

   A. sulfur granules
   B. fat globules
   C. metachromatic granules
   D. Negri bodies
   E. tubercles   (2:323)

11. The dark field illumination method is widely used in the examination of

   A. aerobic bacteria
   B. *M. tuberculosis*
   C. sporozoa
   D. spirochetes
   E. influenza organisms   (2:94)

12. Most pathogenic bacteria grow well at a temperature of approximately

   A. 15°C
   B. 20°C
   C. 25°C
   D. 30°C
   E. 37°C   (2:78)

13. The most common cause of severe infections in hospitals is

   A. *Mycobacterium tuberculosis*
   B. *Escherichia coli*
   C. *Streptococcus fecalis*
   D. *Staphylococcus aureus*
   E. *Staphylococcus albus*   (2:292)

14. Streptococci that hemolyze red blood cells and produce colonies on blood agar surrounded by clear zones are called the

   A. alpha type
   B. beta type
   C. C-type
   D. O-type
   E. *Staphylococcus albus*   (2:296)

15. Dermatomycosis is caused by

   A. protozoa

B. viruses
C. fungi
D. rickettsiae
E. none of the above   (2:484)

16. A disease transmitted by mosquitoes is

   A. typhoid fever
   B. measles
   C. mumps
   D. tuberculosis
   E. yellow fever   (2:465)

17. Negri bodies are cytoplasmic inclusions associated with

   A. rabies
   B. hepatitus
   C. yellow fever
   D. mumps
   E. chickenpox   (2:459)

18. An example of a contagious disease is

   A. common cold
   B. hemophilia
   C. appendicitis
   D. glaucoma
   E. cataract   (2:456)

19. Of the following diseases, the one that is communicable is

   A. anemia
   B. peptic ulcer
   C. tuberculosis
   D. cancer
   E. cataract   (2:456)

20. The phenol coefficient is generally used in the

   A. standardization of disinfectants
   B. analysis of food
   C. analysis of the gastric fluid
   D. study of antibiotics
   E. study of blood groups   (2:241)

21. Vaccination can be used to control

   A. anemia
   B. arthritis
   C. malaria

D. poliomyelitis
E. all of the above   (2:595)

22. BCG vaccine is used to protect against

    A. tuberculosis
    B. rheumatic fever
    C. tetanus
    D. diphtheria
    E. rabies   (2:591)

23. The incubation period for syphilis is approximately

    A. one day
    B. 72 hours
    C. one week
    D. 2 to 6 weeks
    E. 3 to 4 months   (2:402)

24. The predominant organism in milk and the chief cause of its souring is

    A. *Lactobacillus casei*
    B. *Streptococcus lactis*
    C. *Streptococcus bovis*
    D. *Lactobacillus brevis*
    E. *Sarcina lutea*   (2:574)

25. All of the following diseases can be transmitted to man from contaminated milk except

    A. tularemia
    B. diphtheria
    C. scarlet fever
    D. septic sore throat
    E. brucellosis   (2:570)

26. Contaminated milk may transmit

    A. typhoid fever
    B. septic sore throat
    C. diphtheria
    D. scarlet fever
    E. all of the above   (2:570)

27. A bacterial capsule is well developed in

    A. *Diplococcus pneumoniae*
    B. *Clostridium perfringens*
    C. *Klebsiella pneumoniae*
    D. all of the above
    E. none of the above   (2:67)

28. Doctor Jonas Salk discovered a vaccine for the prevention of

    A. poliomyelitis
    B. tetanus
    C. smallpox
    D. measles
    E. yellow fever   (2:35)

29. Doctor Edward Jenner

    A. was an English physician
    B. made the first vaccine for smallpox
    C. lived at the end of the eighteenth century
    D. all of the above
    E. none of the above   (2:19)

30. Lockjaw is a synonym for

    A. rabies
    B. leprosy
    C. leptospirosis
    D. varicella
    E. tetanus   (2:334)

31. Tetanus

    A. is also called lockjaw
    B. is a very serious disease
    C. is caused by anaerobic organisms
    D. all of the above
    E. none of the above   (2:334)

32. *Clostridium botulinum* may cause

    A. meningitis
    B. osteomyelitis
    C. sinusitis
    D. food poisoning
    E. urinary tract infections   (2:338)

33. The cause of human tuberculosis was discovered by

    A. Jonas Salk
    B. Louis Pasteur
    C. Robert Koch
    D. Joseph Lister
    E. none of the above   (2:23)

34. *Coxiella burnetii* causes

    A. Saint Louis encephalitis
    B. Q fever
    C. trench fever
    D. murine typhus
    E. Pappataci fever   (2:420)

35. An attenuated virus can be used to prevent

    A. osteoarthritis
    B. malaria
    C. rheumatoid arthritis
    D. smallpox
    E. all of the above   (2:597)

36. Myxoviruses cause

    A. mumps
    B. measles
    C. dengue fever
    D. vaccinia
    E. herpes zoster   (2:429)

37. The ECHO virus may cause

    A. acute upper respiratory disease
    B. diarrheal disease
    C. aseptic meningitis
    D. exanthematous disease
    E. all of the above   (2:453)

38. All of the following are viral diseases *except*

    A. yellow fever
    B. mumps
    C. influenza
    D. actinomycosis
    E. polio   (2:494)

39. Arborviruses can cause

    A. trachoma
    B. measles
    C. smallpox
    D. yellow fever
    E. herpes simplex   (2:429)

40. Papova viruses cause

    A. chickenpox
    B. influenza
    C. warts

    D. rabies
    E. measles   (2:428)

41. The incubation period of smallpox is

    A. 2 days
    B. 4 days
    C. 12 days
    D. 3 weeks
    E. 5 weeks   (2:447)

42. Lymphogranuloma venereum is

    A. also called climatic bubo
    B. a viral desease
    C. transmitted by venereal contact
    D. all of the above
    E. none of the above   (2:468)

43. *Aedes aegypti* is the vector in

    A. yellow fever
    B. malaria
    C. trench fever
    D. murine typhus
    E. Q fever   (2:465)

44. The incubation period for measles is

    A. 2 to 5 days
    B. 6 to 8 days
    C. 10 to 14 days
    D. 3 weeks
    E. 5 weeks   (2:472)

45. The incubation period of mumps is

    A. 3 to 4 days
    B. 5 to 8 days
    C. 10 to 12 days
    D. 18 to 21 days
    E. 30 days   (2:472)

46. The habitat of *Ascaris lumbricoides* is the

    A. cecum
    B. sigmoid
    C. appendix
    D. small intestine
    E. liver   (2:526)

47. Urinary bilharziasis is caused by

    A. *Schistosoma haematobium*

B. *Schistosoma japonicum*
C. *Schistosoma mansoni*
D. *Paragonimus westermani*
E. none of the above   (2:515)

48. Pinworm infection is caused by

A. ascaris
B. *Trichuris dispar*
C. *Enterobius vermicularis*
D. *Wuchereria bancrofti*
E. *Taenia solium*   (2:526)

49. *Trypanosoma cruzi* is the cause of

A. dumdum fever
B. oriental sore
C. forest yaws
D. Chaga's disease
E. uta   (2:504)

50. The cause of histoplasmosis is a/an

A. virus
B. fungus
C. parasite
D. spirochete
E. acid-fast organism   (2:459)

51. Erythrasma is caused by

A. *Penicillium mucor*
B. *Nocardia tenuis*
C. *Piedraia hortai*
D. *Corynebacterium minutissimum*
E. *Trichosporon beigelii*   (2:493)

52. *Torula histolytica*

A. is a synonym for *Cryptococcus neoformans*
B. is a true yeast
C. reproduces by budding
D. produces sporadic infections
E. all of the above   (2:490,491)

53. Hansen's bacillus causes

A. tuberculosis
B. leprosy
C. trachoma
D. pertussis
E. none of the above   (2:387)

54. Scarlet fever is caused by

A. streptococcus
B. staphylococcus
C. pneumococcus
D. *Clostridium novyi*
E. *Clostridium septicum*   (2:301)

55. Pneumococcus

A. is acid-fast
B. is motile
C. is spore-forming
D. all of the above
E. none of the above   (2:305,306)

56. The following are narrow-spectrum antibiotics *except*

A. erthyromycin
B. vancomycin
C. kanamycin
D. penicillin
E. colistin   (2:255)

57. Antibiotics which act through inhibition of protein synthesis include

A. streptomycin
B. chloramphenicol
C. erythromycin
D. neomycin
E. all of the above   (2:256)

58. *Corynebacterium diphtheriae*

A. is gram-negative
B. is a slender rod-shaped organism
C. ferments sucrose
D. all of the above
E. none of the above   (2:323)

59. The Shigella organisms

A. are gram-negative
B. grow best under aerobic conditions
C. ferment carbohydrates
D. all of the above
E. none of the above   (2:350,351)

60. *Salmonella typhosa*

A. does not produce indole
B. ferments lactose

C. does not stain with ordinary aniline dyes
D. is spore-forming
E. all of the above   (2:344)

61. Hansen's bacillus is also called

A. *Treponema pallidum*
B. *N. gonorrheae*
C. *E. coli*
D. *Mycobacterium tuberculosis*
E. *Mycobacterium leprae*   (2:387)

62. Woolsorter's disease is caused by

A. virus
B. *Streptococcus bovis*
C. *Bacillus anthracis*
D. neisseria
E. pneumococcus   (2:331)

Answer the questions in this group by following the directions below. Select

A. **if only A is correct**
B. **if only B is correct**
C. **if both A and B are correct**
D. **if both A and B are incorrect**

63. Methods used for the study of bacteria include

A. culture
B. direct examination of smears
C. both
D. neither   (2:92,101)

64. A toxin

A. is a substance produced by bacteria
B. is always harmless
C. both
D. neither   (2:87)

65. Milk pasteurization

A. destroys disease organisms
B. increases the fat content of the milk
C. both
D. neither   (2:570)

66. Louis Pasteur

A. is called the father of bacteriology
B. discovered that microbes can cause disease
C. both
D. neither   (2:21)

67. Food poisoning can be caused by

A. Salmonella organisms
B. staphylococcus organisms
C. both
D. neither   (2:576)

68. Pasteurization

A. was named after Louis Pasteur
B. is a process which destroys all pathogenic bacteria
C. both
D. neither   (2:21)

69. Malaria

A. is a disease caused by protozoa
B. is transmitted to man through the bite of the anopheles mosquito
C. both
D. neither   (2:506)

70. Amoebae

A. use pseudopodia for motion
B. may cause scarlet fever
C. both
D. neither   (2:503)

71. Malaria

A. is caused by a virus
B. is less dangerous than chickenpox
C. both
D. neither   (2:506)

72. Smallpox

A. is caused by a virus
B. is less dangerous than chickenpox
C. both
D. neither   (2:473)

73. Infectious mononucleosis

A. is more common in infants

B. is a benign disease
C. both
D. neither   (2:473)

74. Chickenpox

    A. is a viral disease
    B. is also called varicella
    C. both
    D. neither   (2:448)

75. Tuberculosis

    A. is caused by an acid-fast bacillus
    B. can be cured with emetine hyd-
       rochloride
    C. both
    D. neither   (2:374)

76. Leprosy

    A. is caused by an organism discovered by
       Hansen
    B. can be treated with sodium diazone
    C. both
    D. neither   (2:387)

77. Tetanus

    A. is caused by gram-positive rods that
       form spores
    B. is also called "lockjaw"
    C. both
    D. neither   (2:334,335)

78. Diseases caused by spirochetes include

    A. yaws
    B. relapsing fever
    C. both
    D. neither   (2:408,409)

79. Antibodies appearing in the serum after syphilitic infection include

    A. erythrogenic toxin
    B. reagin
    C. both
    D. neither   (2:405)

80. Weil's disease

    A. is caused by *Leptospira icterohaemor-rhagiae*

B. is associated with jaundice
C. both
D. neither   (2:409)

81. Yaws

    A. does not occur in the congenital form
    B. is a venereal disease
    C. both
    D. neither   (2:408)

82. Ringworm of the groin is known as

    A. tinea cruris
    B. dhobie itch
    C. both
    D. neither   (2:485)

83. Metachromatic granules

    A. are enzymatically active
    B. are found in the anthrax bacillus
    C. both
    D. neither   (2:68)

84. Infectious hepatitis

    A. is found only in man
    B. differs epidemiologically from serum
       hepatitis
    C. both
    D. neither   (2:469)

85. BCG vaccine

    A. is administered superficially into the
       skin of the upper arm
    B. is advised for children in areas where
       tuberculosis is a major health problem
    C. both
    D. neither   (2:)

86. *Clostridium perfringens*

    A. causes food poisoning
    B. is also called *Clostridium welchii*
    C. both
    D. neither   (2:337)

87. *Clostridium tetani* ferments

    A. glucose
    B. sucrose

C. both
D. neither   (2:337)

88. *Clostridium botulinum* ferments

   A. lactose
   B. glucose
   C. both
   D. neither   (2:337)

89. *Clostridium novyi* is

   A. spore-forming
   B. motile
   C. both
   D. neither   (2:337)

90. *Clostridium botulinum*

   A. is anaerobic
   B. is gram-positive
   C. both
   D. neither   (2:339)

91. *Clostridium septicum*

   A. ferments glucose and lactose
   B. is motile
   C. both
   D. neither   (2:337)

92. Live, attenuated measles virus vaccines should *not* be given to patients suffering from

   A. leukemia
   B. lymphoma
   C. both
   D. neither   (2:616)

93. *Mycobacterium leprae* is

   A. acid-fast
   B. gram-negative
   C. both
   D. neither   (2:387,388)

94. Flea-borne typhus includes

   A. Rocky Mountain spotted fever
   B. scrub typhus
   C. both
   D. neither   (2:415)

95. Chigger-borne typhus includes

   A. scrub typhus
   B. rickettsial pox
   C. both
   D. neither   (2:415)

96. Rickettsial pox is

   A. a louse-born infection
   B. caused by *Rickettsia akari*
   C. both
   D. neither   (2:488)

97. Louse-borne typhus includes

   A. trench fever
   B. murine endemic typhus
   C. both
   D. neither   (2:415)

98. Pathogenic Rickettsiae include

   A. *Rickettsia rickettsii*
   B. *Rickettsia akari*
   C. both
   D. neither   (2:415)

99. Rickettsial diseases are vectored by

   A. ticks
   B. lice
   C. both
   D. neither   (2:415)

100. Rickettsiae are

   A. gram-positive
   B. extracellular parasites
   C. both
   D. neither   (2:414)

101. *Coxiella burnetti*

   A. produces a rash in infected persons
   B. is not transmitted to man by an insect vector
   C. both
   D. neither   (2:420)

102. Diseases caused by viruses include

   A. poliomyelitis

B. malaria
C. both
D. neither   (2:462)

103. Interferon is

A. a protein
B. nonantigenic
C. both
D. neither   (2:435,436)

104. Hoof-and-mouth disease

A. is caused by fungus
B. rarely causes human infections
C. both
D. neither   (2:473)

105. Dengue fever is

A. a mosquito-borne virus disease
B. characterized by a skin rash
C. both
D. neither   (2:466)

106. Protozoa

A. consist of single cells
B. are usually larger than fungi
C. both
D. neither   (2:498)

107. Diseases caused by protozoa include

A. sleeping sickness
B. amoebic dysentery
C. both
D. neither   (2:502,503)

108. Pathogenic trypanosomes found in man include

A. *Trypanosoma gambiense*
B. *Trypanosoma cruzi*
C. both
D. neither   (2:504)

109. Kala-azar is

A. caused by *Leishmania tropica*
B. also called espundia
C. both
D. neither   (2:505)

110. Dermatophyte species include

A. *Trichophyton rubrum*
B. *Candida albicans*
C. both
D. neither   (2:406,489)

111. Complement-fixing antibodies can be found in patients with

A. syphilis
B. coccidioidomycosis
C. both
D. neither   (2:183,489)

112. *Histoplasma capsulatum*

A. causes Darling's disease
B. is a dimorphic fungus
C. both
D. neither   (2:489)

113. Conditions caused by fungi include

A. favus
B. enterobiasis
C. both
D. neither   (2:485)

114. *Cryptococcus neoformans* is

A. a true yeast
B. also known as *Torula histolytica*
C. both
D. neither   (2:491)

115. Toxic products of streptococci include

A. erythrogenic toxin
B. streptodornase
C. both
D. neither   (2:298)

116. Anaerobic bacteria

A. live in the absence of free oxygen
B. can obtain their oxygen from the chemical compounds on which they grow
C. both
D. neither   (2:79)

117. Endotoxins

A. are lipopolysaccharides

B. are related to the cell wall of most gram-negative bacteria
C. both
D. neither   (2:87)

118. Transduction

A. involves the transfer of bits of genetic material from bacterium to bacterium
B. occurs in certain enteric pathogens
C. both
D. neither   (2:75)

119. Broad-spectrum antibiotics include

A. ampicillin
B. novobiocin
C. both
D. neither   (2:255)

120. Penicillin is

A. bactericidal
B. the first antibiotic to come into general use
C. both
D. neither   (2:258)

121. Fumagillin is destructive to

A. *Entamoeba histolytica*
B. most fungi
C. both
D. neither   (2:262)

122. Diphtheria bacilli are

A. resistant to drying
B. easily destroyed by heat
C. both
D. neither   (2:324)

123. *Corynebacterium diphtheriae* ferments

A. sucrose
B. trehalose
C. both
D. neither   (2:329)

124. Shigellae fermenting mannitol include

A. *Shigella sonnei*
B. *Shigella dysenteriae*

C. both
D. neither   (2:354)

125. *Escherichia coli*

A. produces indol
B. gives a negative Voges-Proskauer reaction
C. both
D. neither   (2:354)

126. *Aerobacter aerogenes* gives

A. a negative methyl red reaction
B. a positive Voges-Proskauer reaction
C. both
D. neither   (2:354)

127. Antigens identified in *Salmonella typhosa* include

A. O or somatic group antigen
B. H or flagellar specific antigen
C. both
D. neither   (2:348)

128. Typhoid fever

A. is milder than paratyphoid fever
B. has a shorter duration than paratyphoid fever
C. both
D. neither   (2:349)

129. Abert's stain uses

A. toluidine blue
B. malachite green
C. both
D. neither   (2:99)

130. The Kahn test for syphilis

A. is a complement fixation test
B. is used for screening sera because it is relatively quick and simple
C. both
D. neither   (2:406)

131. Negative Weil-Felix reaction is seen in

A. Q fever

B. epidemic typhus
C. both
D. neither   (2:415)

132. Acid-fast organisms encountered in medicine include

   A. *Mycobacterium tuberculosis*
   B. *Nocardia asteroides*
   C. both
   D. neither   (2:99)

133. Indole-producing bacteria include

   A. proteus
   B. *Escherichia coli*
   C. both
   D. neither   (2:118)

Each statement is followed by four suggested answers. Answer according to the following key:

   A. if answers 1, 2, and 3 are correct
   B. if 1 and 3 are correct
   C. if 2 and 4 are correct
   D. if only 4 is correct
   E. if all are correct

134. Stains designed to demonstrate metachromatic granules are especially valuable in identifying

   1. *Treponema pallidum*
   2. *Streptococcus viridans*
   3. *Streptococcus lactis*
   4. *Corynebacterium diphtheriae*   (2:99)

135. Albert's stain uses

   1. toluidine blue
   2. methylene blue
   3. malachite green
   4. carbolfuchsin   (2:99)

136. Gram-negative cocci include

   1. *Streptococcus pyogenes*
   2. *Neisseria gonorrheae*
   3. *Staphylococcus aureus*
   4. *Neisseria meningitidis*   (2:97)

137. Gram-negative bacilli include

   1. *Salmonella typhosa*
   2. *Mycobacterium leprae*
   3. *Haemophilus influenzae*
   4. *Bacillus anthracis*   (2:97)

138. Gram-positive bacteria include

   1. *Clostridium tetani*
   2. *Neisseria gonorrheae*
   3. *Mycobacterium tuberculosis*
   4. *Escherichia coli*   (2:97)

139. The Ziehl-Neelsen stain is

   1. a spore stain
   2. a capsule stain
   3. a flagella stain
   4. an acid-fast stain   (2:98)

140. Hyaluronidase

   1. is a pigment
   2. is produced by pneumococci
   3. is an endos toxin
   4. changes the consistency of tissues
                                     (2:90)

141. Spore formation is characteristic of

   1. spirochetes
   2. cocci
   3. vibriones
   4. bacilli   (2:71)

142. Toxins

   1. are protein in composition
   2. are antigenic
   3. are specific
   4. stimulate the production of antitoxins when injected into an animal   (2:87)

143. Food poisoning may be caused by

   1. *Proteus vulgaris*
   2. *Clostridium botulinum*
   3. *Taenia saginata*
   4. *Staphylococci*   (2:576)

144. Laboratory aids in the diagnosis of brucellosis include

   1. an agglutination test
   2. positive Kveim test

3. positive blood culture
4. positive Wasserman test (2:366)

145. Brucellosis is contracted from
    1. mosquitoes
    2. mice
    3. dogs
    4. cattle (2:366)

146. The common form of brucellosis is characterized by
    1. fever
    2. marked weakness
    3. profuse sweating
    4. convulsions (2:365)

147. Torulosis
    1. is also called Gilchrist's disease
    2. may cause thickening of the meninges
    3. is caused by *Candida albicans*
    4. is fungal disease (2:490)

148. *Cryptococcus neoformans* has been found in
    1. cattle
    2. horses
    3. dogs
    4. cats (2:490)

149. Yellow fever
    1. is a mosquito-borne disease
    2. has an abrupt onset
    3. has a rapid course
    4. causes extensive destruction of the liver (2:465)

150. Prominent symptoms of yellow fever include
    1. jaundice
    2. vomiting
    3. hemorrhage
    4. albumin in the urine (2:465)

151. Dengue fever
    1. is also called "breakbone fever"
    2. is a viral disease

3. does not cause skin rash
4. lasts 10 days (2:466)

152. Rabies
    1. is transmitted chiefly by dogs
    2. shows two clinical forms, the furious and the dumb
    3. is transmitted through saliva containing virus
    4. is always fatal once the disease develops (2:457,458)

153. Poliomyelitis
    1. may occur in epidemics, but tends to be sporadic
    2. in its severe form, affects the brain and the spinal cord
    3. inevitably results upon infection with the virus
    4. virus is present in the pharynx and the stools of the patients (2:462)

154. Serum hepatitis
    1. has an acute onset
    2. affects only adults
    3. has a seasonal peak during the winter
    4. has an incubation period of 2 to 6 months (2:470)

155. Trachoma
    1. is one of the oldest diseases
    2. afflicts 500 million persons in the world
    3. is caused by one of the bedsoniae
    4. is associated with characteristic inclusion bodies (2:468)

156. Live attenuated measles virus vaccines should not be given to patients treated with
    1. steroids
    2. irradiation
    3. antimetabolites
    4. agents that depress the individuals immunologic capacities (2:616)

157. Influenza vaccination is recommended for

    1. persons over 65 years of age
    2. residents of nursing homes
    3. individuals with chronic debilitating diseases
    4. law enforcement officers   (2:612)

158. Mumps

    1. is also called epidemic parotitis
    2. is an acute disease
    3. is caused by a virus in the myxovirus group
    4. occurs more often between the second and third years   (2:471)

159. *Escherichia coli*

    1. is gram-negative
    2. does not form spores
    3. grows best at 37°C
    4. is a normal inhabitant of the intestinal tract   (2:353)

160. Pasteurization of milk

    1. involves heating it below the boiling point
    2. does not change its compostion
    3. kills all nonspore-bearing, disease-producing bacteria
    4. kills all nonspore-bearing, non-pathogenic bacteria   (2:233)

161. Antiseptics and disinfectants act by

    1. hydrolysis
    2. coagulation of proteins
    3. oxidation of the microbial cell
    4. disruption of the microbial cell(2:239)

162. *Tinea capitis*

    1. is also called ringworm of the scalp
    2. is caused by fungi
    3. is caused by trichophyton
    4. is treated with penicillin   (2:484)

163. Farm animals may be a source of which of the following infections?

    1. ornithosis
    2. salmonellosis
    3. brucellosis
    4. tuberculosis   (2:164)

164. Rodents may be a source of which of the following infections?

    1. tularemia
    2. toxoplasmosis
    3. leptospirosis
    4. roundworm infection   (2:164)

165. Dogs may be a source of which of the following infections?

    1. rabies
    2. anthrax
    3. ringworm
    4. scabies   (2:164)

166. Cats may be a source of which of the following infections?

    1. cat scratch disease
    2. psittacosis
    3. rabies
    4. encephalitis   (2:164)

167. Man may acquire an infectious disease by

    1. direct contact with an infected animal
    2. insect vectors
    3. contaminated air
    4. contaminated water   (2:163)

168. Water-borne diseases include

    1. plague
    2. salmonellosis
    3. aspergillosis
    4. amoebic dysentery   (2:561)

169. Water-borne diseases include

    1. viral hepatitis
    2. erysipelas
    3. cholera
    4. yellow fever   (2:561)

Directions: Each group of numbered words and statements is followed by the same number of lettered words, phrases or statements. For each numbered word or statement choose the lettered item that is most closely related to it.

Questions 170 to 174

170. Developed the tuberculin test
171. Discovered the blood groups
172. Discovered penicillin
173. Discovered a vaccine for polio
174. Discovered drugs against syphilis

    A. Robert Koch
    B. Paul Ehrlich
    C. Landsteiner
    D. Fleming
    E. Salk   (2:23,29,30,35)

Questions 175 to 179

175. Theodore Schwann
176. Edward Jenner
177. Joseph Lister
178. Louis Pasteur
179. Alphonse Laveran

    A. Introduced vaccination to prevent smallpox
    B. Proved that yeasts are living things
    C. Developed anthrax
    D. Applied antiseptic treatment to the prevention of wound infections
    E. Discovered the parasite of malaria   (2:19,21,22,23)

Questions 180 to 184

180. Developed with Gengou the process of complement fixation
181. Discovered diphtheria toxin
182. Discribed *Treponema pallidum,* the causative agent of syphilis
183. Announced the phagocytic theory of immunity
184. Determined the value of penicillin as a theurapeutic agent

    A. Roux
    B. Elie Metchnikoff
    C. Bordet
    D. Schaudin
    E. Florey   (2:23,26,28,29,31)

Questions 185 to 188

185. Discovered tyrothricin
186. Discovered streptomycin
187. Developed the oral poliovirus vaccine
188. Established the value of Prontosil in streptococcal infections

    A. Domagk
    B. René Dubos
    C. Waksman
    D. Albert Sabin   (2:31,32,34)

Questions 189 to 192

189. 7 to 14 days' incubation period
190. 2 to 6 days' incubation period
191. 5 to 21 days' incubation period
192. 8 to 10 weeks' incubation period

    A. Diphtheria
    B. Mycoplasmal pneumonia
    C. Pertussis
    D. Tapeworm infections   (2:158)

Questions 193 to 196

193. 7 to 21 days' incubation period
194. 2 to 10 weeks' incubation period
195. 1 to 10 days' incubation period
196. 6 to 48 hours' incubation period

    A. Food poisoning (salmonellosis)
    B. Paratyphoid fever
    C. Typhoid fever
    D. Tuberculosis (primary lesion) (2:158)

Questions 197 to 201

197. 3 to 5 days' incubation period
198. 14 to 16 days' incubation period
199. 3 to 6 weeks' incubation period
200. 1 to 3 days' incubation period
201. 14 to 28 days' incubation period

    A. Influenza
    B. Gonorrhea
    C. Chickenpox
    D. Mumps
    E. Pinworm infection   (2:158)

Questions 202 to 206

202. 14 to 22 days' incubation period
203. 7 to 14 days' incubation period
204. 1 to 4 days' incubation period
205. 15 to 40 days' incubation period

206. 45 to 160 days' incubation period

    A. Dysentery caused by Shigellae
    B. Herpes zoster
    C. Infectious hepatitis
    D. Serum hepatitis
    E. Rubella   (2:350,445,448,470)

Questions 207 to 211

207. Sarcoidosis
208. Tularemia
209. Hydatid disease
210. Syphilis
211. Diphtheria

    A. Wasserman test
    B. Schick test
    C. Foshay test
    D. Casoni's test
    E. Kveim test   (2:329,371,405)

Questions 212 to 216

212. Typhoid fever
213. Tuberculosis
214. Scarlet fever
215. Typhus
216. Infectious mononucleosis

    A. Weil-Felix test
    B. Widal test
    C. Mantoux test
    D. Paul Bunnel test
    E. Dick test   (2:182,302,347,383,415)

Questions 217 to 220

217. Lymphogranuloma venereum
218. Syphilis
219. Scarlet fever
220. Used to detect the absence of antibodies against pneumococci
221. Used to detect sensitivity to diphtheria toxoid

    A. Frei test
    B. Schultz-Charlton test
    C. Kahn test
    D. Francis test
    E. Maloney test   (2:28,302,468)

Questions 222 to 226

222. May be transmitted by mosquitoes
223. Ulcerative condition of the throat
224. May cause orchitis
225. Dangerous in pregnant women
226. "Black death"

    A. German measles
    B. Mumps
    C. Yellow fever
    D. Bubonic plague
    E. Vincent's angina (2:370,445,465,473)

Questions 227 to 231

227. Dwarf tapeworm
228. Dog tapeworm
229. Pork tapeworm
230. Beef tapeworm
231. Fish tapeworm

    A. *Taenia solium*
    B. *Taenia saginata*
    C. *Hymenolepis nana*
    D. *Diphyllobothrium latum*
    E. *Dipylidium caninum* (2:519,520,521)

Questions 232 to 235

232. *Clostridium tetani*
233. Staphylococcus
234. *Clostridium perfringens*
235. Streptococcus

    A. Cause of furuncles
    B. Cause of Scarlet fever
    C. Cause of lockjaw
    D. Cause of gas gangrene
               (2:291,301,334,337,350)

Questions 236 to 240

236. *Vibrio comma*
237. *Salmonella typhosa*
238. *Escherichia coli*
239. Friedlander's bacillus
240. Bordet-Gengou bacillus

    A. Cause of typhoid fever
    B. Cause of cholera
    C. Can cause pneumonia
    D. Can cause pyelonephritis
    E. Causes pertussis
            (2:345,352,355,356,360)

Questions 241 to 245

241. Trichophyton
242. Coxsackie virus
243. Epidermophyton
244. *Cryptococcus neoformans*
245. *Histoplasma capsulatum*

    A. May cause epidemic pleurodynia
    B. May cause ringworm of the scalp
    C. May cause ringworm of the body
    D. Causes Darling's disease
    E. Causes torulosis (2:464,484,489,490)

Questions 246 to 250

246. *Leishmania braziliensis*
247. *Candida albicans*
248. *Leishmania donovoni*
249. Penicillium
250. *Nocardia minutissima*

    A. Cause of moniliasis
    B. Cause of otomycosis
    C. Cause of erythrasma
    D. Cause of kala-azar
    E. Cause of espundia   (2:491,493,505)

Answer Key: Microbiology

1. A	33. C	65. A	97. A	129. C	161. E	193. C	225. A
2. C	34. B	66. C	98. C	130. B	162. A	194. D	226. D
3. B	35. D	67. C	99. C	131. A	163. E	195. B	227. C
4. A	36. A	68. C	100. D	132. C	164. B	196. A	228. E
5. C	37. A	69. C	101. B	133. C	165. E	197. B	229. A
6. A	38. D	70. A	102. A	134. D	166. B	198. C	230. B
7. E	39. D	71. D	103. C	135. B	167. E	199. E	231. D
8. C	40. C	72. A	104. B	136. C	168. C	200. A	232. C
9. C	41. C	73. B	105. C	137. B	169. B	201. D	233. A
10. C	42. D	74. C	106. A	138. B	170. A	202. E	234. D
11. D	43. A	75. A	107. C	139. D	171. C	203. B	235. B
12. E	44. C	76. C	108. C	140. C	172. D	204. A	236. B
13. D	45. D	77. C	109. D	141. B	173. E	205. C	237. A
14. B	46. D	78. C	110. A	142. E	174. B	206. D	238. D
15. C	47. A	79. B	111. C	143. C	175. B	207. E	239. C
16. E	48. C	80. C	112. C	144. B	176. A	208. C	240. E
17. A	49. D	81. A	113. A	145. D	177. D	209. D	241. B
18. A	50. B	82. C	114. C	146. A	178. C	210. A	242. A
19. C	51. D	83. A	115. C	147. C	179. E	211. B	243. C
20. A	52. E	84. C	116. C	148. E	180. C	212. B	244. E
21. D	53. B	85. C	117. C	149. E	181. A	213. C	245. D
22. A	54. A	86. B	118. C	150. E	182. D	214. E	246. E
23. D	55. E	87. D	119. A	151. C	183. B	215. A	247. A
24. B	56. C	88. B	120. C	152. E	184. E	216. D	248. D
25. A	57. E	89. C	121. A	153. C	185. B	217. A	249. B
26. E	58. B	90. C	122. C	154. D	186. C	218. C	250. C
27. D	59. D	91. C	123. D	155. E	187. D	219. B	
28. A	60. A	92. C	124. A	156. E	188. A	220. D	
29. D	61. E	93. A	125. C	157. E	189. B	221. E	
30. E	62. C	94. D	126. C	158. A	190. A	222. C	
31. D	63. C	95. A	127. C	159. E	191. C	223. E	
32. D	64. A	96. B	128. D	160. E	192. D	224. B	

Chapter Three

Pharmacology

Directions: Select from among the lettered choices the one that most appropriately answers the question or completes the statement.

1. Of the following agents, the one that produces a persistent increase in plasma volume is
   A. dextran
   B. dextrose solution
   C. saline
   D. norepinephrine
   E. ephedrine   (3:182)

2. Drugs that make the skin and the mucous membranes constrict are called
   A. carminatives
   B. caustics
   C. astringents
   D. ecbolics
   E. emollients   (3:55)

3. A drug that relieves swelling of the nasal mucosa is a
   A. demulcent
   B. decongestant
   C. depilatory
   D. digestant
   E. hydragogue   (3:335)

4. Side effects of Levodopa include
   A. phlebitis
   B. hypertension
   C. opisthotonos
   D. all of the above
   E. none of the above   (3:399)

5. Respiratory stimulation can be induced by
   A. Coramine
   B. Dopram
   C. Emivan
   D. Megimide
   E. all of the above   (3:330,331)

6. The main use of streptomycin is in the treatment of
   A. rheumatic fever
   B. typhoid fever
   C. tuberculosis
   D. osteomyelitis
   E. none of the above   (3:581)

7. Mandelamine is used as
   A. a urinary antiseptic
   B. an expectorant
   C. a cardiac stimulant
   D. a sedative
   E. an emetic   (3:216)

8. Examples of central nervous system stimulants include
   A. amphetamine
   B. ephedrine
   C. niketamide
   D. all of the above
   E. none of the above   (3:274)

9. Anticholinergic agents
   A. relax smooth muscles
   B. dilate the pupils

C. inhibit secretions of duct glands
D. compete with acetylcholine
E. all of the above   (3:121)

10. Veratrum products are contraindicated in patients with

A. uremia
B. digitalis intoxication
C. cerebrovascular disease
D. all of the above
E. none of the above   (3:167)

11. Benzocaine is a

A. general anesthetic
B. sedative
C. local anesthetic
D. diuretic
E. purgative   (3:317)

12. The *least* toxic of all local anesthetic drugs is

A. procaine
B. cocaine
C. xylocaine
D. carbocaine
E. pontocaine   (3:316)

13. Which of the following anesthetics is nonflammable?

A. chloroform
B. ether
C. cyclopropane
D. ethyl chloride
E. fluoromar   (3:304)

14. Which of the following is *not* an antibiotic?

A. streptomycin
B. penicillin
C. aureomycin
D. quinidine
E. achromycin   (3:150)

15. The usual oral dose of paraldehyde is

A. 2 ml
B. 5 ml

C. 0.1 ml
D. 10 to 20 ml
E. 30 ml   (3:280)

16. Benemid is useful in the treatment of gout because it

A. decreases uric acid production
B. decreases uric acid excretion
C. increases uric acid excretion
D. alleviates pain
E. none of the above   (3:265)

17. The administration of atropine results in

A. mydriasis - dilate
B. excessive salivation
C. bronchial spasm
D. all of the above
E. none of the above   (3:121)

18. Sulfonamides are indicated in the treatment of

A. trachoma
B. chancroid
C. nocardiosis
D. toxoplasmosis
E. all of the above   (3:561)

19. The duration of action of NPH insulin is

A. 28 to 30 hours
B. 30 to 35 hours
C. 2 to 4 hours
D. 10 to 20 hours   (3:477)

20. An example of a stimulant drug is

A. Coramine
B. chloral hydrate
C. paraldehyde
D. Nembutal
E. Dilantin   (3:274)

21. Pronestyl is

A. effective in cardiac arrhythmias
B. a weak anesthetic
C. used in atrial tachycardia
D. all of the above
E. none of the above   (3:153)

22. Side effects of veratrum alkaloids include

    A. chest pain
    B. vomiting
    C. hiccough
    D. cardiac irregularities
    E. all of the above   (3:167)

23. Side effects due to the administration of reserpine include

    A. edema
    B. weight gain
    C. peptic ulcer
    D. depression
    E. all of the above   (3:163)

24. Tromexan is a synthetic drug with action similar to

    A. heparin
    B. histamine
    C. dicumarol
    D. cocaine
    E. insulin   (3:188)

25. The usual duration of action of an intravenous dose of heparin is

    A. 1 hour
    B. 2 hours
    C. 2 to 4 hours
    D. 8 hours
    E. 12 hours   (3:188)

26. Overdosage of heparin can be counteracted with

    A. folic acid
    B. lactone
    C. protamine
    D. whole blood
    E. Tromexan   (3:189)

27. A patient receiving ferrous sulfate will undergo a change in the color of the

    A. skin
    B. eyes
    C. urine
    D. feces
    E. hair   (3:176)

28. An example of a diuretic is

    A. scopolamine
    B. ephedrine
    C. codeine
    D. caffeine
    E. papaverine   (3:204)

29. All of the following are diuretics *except*

    A. Diamox
    B. spirolactone
    C. cortisone
    D. chlorothiazide
    E. ethacrynic acid   (3:465)

30. All the following are laxatives *except*

    A. cascara sagrada
    B. aloin
    C. phenolphthalein
    D. dulcolax
    E. peritrate   (3:157)

31. An example of an emetic drug is

    A. syrup of ipecac
    B. kaolin
    C. tincture of opium
    D. castor oil
    E. bisacodyl   (3:420)

32. The usual adult dose of milk of magnesia is

    A. 10 mg
    B. 50 mg
    C. 500 mg
    D. 1 to 4 g
    E. 10 g   (3:418)

33. Ascorbic acid is

    A. vitamin A
    B. vitamin E
    C. vitamin K
    D. vitamin D
    E. vitamin C   (3:450)

34. The vitamin used in the treatment of rickets is

    A. vitamin D
    B. vitamin C
    C. vitamin B_{12}

D. thiamin
E. nicotinic acid   (3:443)

35. The average adult dose of paregoric is

A. 4 cc
B. 2 cc
C. 0.5 cc
D. 15 cc
E. 30 cc   (3:246)

36. The average adult dose of amphetamine is

A. ¼ grain
B. ½ grain
C. 1 grain
D. 10 grains
E. 1/12 grain   (3:237)

37. The average adult dose of laudanum is

A. 0.1 cc
B. 0.6 cc
C. 1 cc
D. 4 cc
E. 12 cc   (3:246)

38. Penicillin is highly effective in

A. syphilis
B. gonorrhea
C. actinomycosis
D. bacterial endocarditis
E. all of the above   (3:571)

39. The average daily maintenance dose of digoxin is

A. 0.25 mg
B. 1.0 mg
C. 1.0 g
D. 5.0 mg
E. none of the above   (3:147)

40. The average daily maintenance dose of digitoxin is

A. 0.2 mg
B. 0.1 mg
C. 0.5 mg
D. 0.1 g
E. 0.2 g   (3:146)

41. All of the following are antihistamines *except*

A. Dramamine
B. Benadryl
C. Phenergan
D. Tromexan
E. Chlor-trimeton   (3:188)

42. The most common side effect of antihistamines is

A. diarrhea
B. leucopenia
C. drowsiness
D. constipation
E. nausea   (3:244)

43. Penicillin is not effective against infections caused by

A. tubercle bacillus
B. fungi
C. true viruses
D. amebiasis
E. all of the above   (3:571)

44. An example of an anticonvulsant drug is

A. tridione
B. cocaine
C. codeine
D. cortisone
E. insulin   (3:290)

45. Dilantin is the brand name for

A. primidone
B. trimethadione
C. diphenylhydantoin
D. paramethadione
E. none of the above   (3:288)

46. The major danger from overdose of the curariform drugs is

A. anuria
B. hypotension
C. hemolysis
D. paralysis of respiration
E. ileus   (3:631)

47. Epinephrine

    A. produces a rise in blood sugar
    B. decreases myocardial contraction
    C. decreases cardiac rate
    D. causes constriction of the urinary bladder
    E. none of the above   (3:104–105)

48. The average duration of a dose of protamine zinc insulin is

    A. 1 hour
    B. 3 to 5 hours
    C. 20 to 24 hours
    D. 12 to 16 hours
    E. 24 to 48 hours   (3:477)

49. Propylthioracil is

    A. a vitamin
    B. a goitrogen
    C. an antibiotic
    D. a hormone
    E. none of the above   (3:461)

50. Peripheral neuritis caused by isoniazid can be prevented if the drug is given together with

    A. pyridoxine
    B. folic acid
    C. thiamine
    D. insulin
    E. niacin   (3:598)

51. A toxic effect that may result from the use of pitocin is

    A. rupture of the uterus
    B. decreased urinary output
    C. respiratory depression
    D. severe hypotension
    E. increased sodium retention   (3:527)

52. The most common side effect in patients receiving reserpine is

    A. stuffiness of the nose
    B. drowsiness
    C. insomnia
    D. tremor of the hands
    E. nausea   (3:163)

53. Dimercaprol is an antidote for which of the following poisons?

    A. antimony
    B. mercury
    C. Fowler's solution
    D. all of the above
    E. none of the above   (3:640)

54. BAL (British Anti-Lewisite) is used to counteract the toxic effects of

    A. mercury
    B. morphine
    C. salicylates
    D. barbiturates
    E. atropine   (6:640)

55. After using a household cleaning compound to remove spots from a dress, a housewife becomes jaundiced. The compound that she used most probably contained

    A. lauryl sulfate
    B. ammonia
    C. benzine
    D. ether
    E. carbon tetrachloride   (3:636)

Answer the questions in this group by following the directions below. Select

    A. if only A is correct
    B. if only B is correct
    C. if both A and B are correct
    D. if both A and B are incorrect

56. Cocaine

    A. is less potent than procaine
    B. can produce surface anesthesia to the eye nose and throat
    C. both
    D. neither   (3:314)

57. Drugs may decrease free norepinephrine in the body by

    A. inhibiting release of norepinephrine
    B. depleting stores of norepinephrine
    C. both
    D. neither   (3:160)

58. Reserpine is administered by

    A. oral route
    B. intramuscular injection
    C. both
    D. neither   (3:163)

59. Poisoning by phenothiazine causes

    A. miosis
    B. irritability
    C. both
    D. neither   (3:629)

60. Pyridium is a

    A. urinary tract antiseptic
    B. cardiac depressant
    C. both
    D. neither   (3:549)

61. Digitalis is contraindicated in

    A. severe myocarditis
    B. heart block
    C. both
    D. neither   (3:147)

62. Tetracycline is

    A. a broad-spectrum antibiotic
    B. the drug of choice in typhoid fever
    C. both
    D. neither   (3:578)

63. Quinine is useful in the treatment of

    A. pinworm infection
    B. ascaris infection
    C. both
    D. neither   (3:602)

64. Amphotericin B is useful in the treatment of

    A. histoplasmosis
    B. malaria
    C. both
    D. neither   (3:590)

65. Coumarin derivatives are

    A. expensive
    B. effective with oral administration

C. both
D. neither   (3:190)

66. Nitrogen mustard is useful in the treatment of

    A. Hodgkin's disease
    B. rheumatoid arthritis
    C. both
    D. neither   (3:501)

67. Procaine is

    A. an anesthetic drug
    B. an anorectic drug
    C. both
    D. neither   (3:316)

68. Procaine is

    A. a local anesthetic
    B. the least toxic of local anesthetics
    C. both
    D. neither   (3:316)

69. Ethyl chloride

    A. is used for topical anesthesia of short duration
    B. acts by freezing the area
    C. both
    D. neither   (3:319)

70. Paraldehyde is a drug with

    A. sedative properties
    B. a disagreeable taste
    C. both
    D. neither   (3:279,280)

71. Barbiturates are used as

    A. sedatives
    B. analeptics
    C. both
    D. neither   (3:269)

72. Paraldehyde

    A. can be given orally
    B. can be given intramuscularly
    C. both
    D. neither   (3:280)

73. The organic mercurial diuretics can be used to relieve edema due to

    A. nephrosis
    B. portal obstruction
    C. both
    D. neither   (3:205)

74. Darvon

    A. is an analgesic drug
    B. produces constipation
    C. both
    D. neither   (3:256,257)

75. An example of an analgesic drug is

    A. Dilantin
    B. dicumarol
    C. both
    D. neither   (3:188,288)

76. Recurrence of acute gout is best prevented by regular administration of

    A. colchicine
    B. gold
    C. both
    D. neither   (3:264)

77. The pharmacological properties of meperidine resemble those of

    A. adrenaline
    B. piperazine
    C. both
    D. neither   (3:250)

78. Morphine causes

    A. dilatation of the pupil
    B. depression of respiration
    C. both
    D. neither   (3:246)

79. Methadone produces

    A. analgesia
    B. addiction
    C. both
    D. neither   (3:251,252)

80. Codeine is

    A. an antipyretic
    B. a miotic
    C. both
    D. neither   (3:247)

81. Iron therapy is used prophylactically in

    A. pregnancy
    B. premature infants
    C. both
    D. neither   (3:174)

82. Apomorphine

    A. is used as an analgesic
    B. has a depressant action on the respiratory center
    C. both
    D. neither   (3:420)

83. Papaverine

    A. has no narcotic effects
    B. is legally classified as a narcotic because it is derived from the opium poppy
    C. both
    D. neither   (3:247)

84. Morphine is an ingredient of

    A. laudanum
    B. paregoric
    C. both
    D. neither   (3:246,248)

85. Morphine is contraindicated for

    A. asthma
    B. head injuries
    C. both
    D. neither   (3:244)

86. Amphetamine

    A. increases the appetite
    B. is a habit-forming drug
    C. both
    D. neither   (3:236)

87. Nalorphine is an antidote against poisoning with

A. morphine
B. strychnine
C. both
D. neither   (3:255)

88. Coramine is

A. a cough depressant
B. an antiemetic drug
C. both
D. neither   (3:331)

89. Mephenesin exhibits a depressant action on the

A. basal ganglia
B. brainstem
C. both
D. neither   (3:396)

90. Cortisone and hydrocortisone are indicated in

A. Addison's disease
B. hypopituitarism
C. both
D. neither   (3:466)

91. The effect of quinidine's action on the electrocardiogram is

A. prolongation of the P-R interval
B. prolongation of QRS duration
C. both
D. neither   (3:151)

92. Nitroglycerin

A. has a long duration of action
B. is usually taken sublingually
C. both
D. neither   (3:157)

93. Ganglionic-blocking antihypertensive drugs include

A. hexamethonium
B. diuril
C. both
D. neither   (3:168)

94. Drugs used in the treatment of hypertension include

A. Aldomet
B. chlorothiazide
C. both
D. neither   (3:165,170)

95. Ismelin

A. is a ganglionic blocker of only the parasympathetic system
B. is used in the treatment of hypertension
C. both
D. neither   (3:164)

96. Side effects due to the administration of ganglionic blocking drugs include

A. excessive salivation
B. difficulty in urination
C. both
D. neither   (3:168)

97. Serpasil

A. contains reserpine
B. is useful in the treatment of hypertension
C. both
D. neither   (3:162,163)

98. Heparin

A. can only be given parenterally
B. is a valuable drug in the treatment of vascular diseases
C. both
D. neither   (3:187)

99. Heparin prolongs the clotting time of blood

A. in the test tube
B. in the blood vessels
C. both
D. neither   (3:187)

100. The major site of action of dicumarol is

A. the blood
B. the liver
C. both
D. neither   (3:189,190)

101. Diuril causes

    A. relief of edema in congestive heart failure
    B. diuresis
    C. both
    D. neither   (3:208)

102. Theophylline is used as a

    A. diuretic
    B. sedative
    C. both
    D. neither   (3:204)

103. Spirolactone

    A. cannot be given orally
    B. increases sodium excretion
    C. both
    D. neither   (3:211)

104. Aldactone

    A. is useful in edema due to liver cirrhosis
    B. antagonizes the action of aldosterone
    C. both
    D. neither   (3:211)

104. A contraindication to the use of ammonium chloride is

    A. cardiac edema
    B. severe kidney disease
    C. both
    D. neither   (3:214)

106. Bacteriostatic antibiotics include

    A. penicillin
    B. streptomycin
    C. both
    D. neither   (3:567)

107. An example of a mercurial diuretic is

    A. Mercuhydrin
    B. Diamox
    C. both
    D. neither   (3:206)

108. An example of an osmotic diuretic is

    A. mannitol
    B. mercaptomerin
    C. both
    D. neither   (3:213)

109. Amphozel acts as

    A. an antiseptic
    B. an antacid
    C. both
    D. neither   (3:415)

110. Saline type laxatives include

    A. magnesium sulfate
    B. mineral oil
    C. both
    D. neither   (3:248)

111. Common antacids include

    A. magnesium trisilicate
    B. milk of magnesia
    C. both
    D. neither   (3:416,418)

112. Dramamine is a

    A. drug for the treatment of vertigo
    B. mydriatic
    C. both
    D. neither   (3:226)

113. Histamine causes

    A. contraction of the uterine muscles
    B. relaxation of the arteries
    C. both
    D. neither   (3:223)

114. Therapeutic uses for histamine include

    A. the common cold
    B. blood transfusion reactions
    C. both
    D. neither   (3:222)

115. Mesantoin is a drug

    A. useful for grand mal epilepsy
    B. that causes gum hypertrophy
    C. both
    D. neither   (3:289)

116. Side effects of treatment with tridione include

    A. diarrhea
    B. sensitivity to light
    C. both
    D. neither   (3:290)

117. Dilantin may cause

    A. hyperplasia of the gums
    B. dermatitis
    C. both
    D. neither   (3:288,289)

118. Toxic effects of Tridione include

    A. hiccup
    B. photophobia
    C. both
    D. neither   (3:290)

119. Toxic effects of Dilantin include

    A. proteinuria
    B. ataxia
    C. both
    D. neither   (3:219)

120. Tensilon is an effective antidote in overdosage of

    A. decamethonium
    B. succinylocholine
    C. both
    D. neither   (3:129)

121. Neostigmine is an effective antidote in overdosage of

    A. tubocurarine
    B. Flaxedil
    C. both
    D. neither   (3:394)

122. Meperidine depresses the central nervous system at

    A. cortical levels
    B. subcortical levels
    C. both
    D. neither   (3:249)

123. Muscle relaxants include

    A. carisoprodol
    B. methocarbamol
    C. both
    D. neither   (3:397)

124. In rheumatoid arthritis, cortisone

    A. may be beneficial in some cases
    B. should always be used
    C. both
    D. neither   (3:466)

125. Cortisone is

    A. derived from the medullary portion of the adrenal glands
    B. an effective anti-inflammatory drug
    C. both
    D. neither   (3:465,466)

126. Prolonged administration of cortisone may cause

    A. loss of hair
    B. "moon" face
    C. both
    D. neither   (3:468)

127. Aldosterone

    A. is formed at the adrenal cortex
    B. promotes the excretion of sodium
    C. both
    D. neither   (3:465)

128. Epinephrine

    A. increases the blood pressure
    B. is used in the treatment of myasthenia gravis
    C. both
    D. neither   (3:104)

129. Thiouracil causes

    A. hyperthyroidism
    B. an increase in basal metabolism
    C. both
    D. neither   (3:461)

130. Symptoms indicating cumulative effects of digitoxin include

A. vomiting
B. visual disturbances
C. both
D. neither   (3:147)

131. Cortisone has

A. antipyretic properties
B. mood-elevating properties
C. both
D. neither   (3:466)

132. The serious toxic effect of chloramphenicol is

A. aplastic anemia
B. dermatitis
C. both
D. neither   (3:584)

133. Signs of nephrotoxicity can be seen following the use of

A. erythromycin
B. streptomycin
C. both
D. neither   (3:581,582)

134. Toxic effects from streptomycin include

A. vestibular damage
B. renal damage
C. both
D. neither   (3:582)

135. Toxic effects from the salicylates include

A. skin rash
B. dry mouth
C. both
D. neither   (3:260)

136. Toxic doses of ergotamine produce

A. sedation
B. peripheral vascular spasm
C. both
D. neither   (3:526)

137. Flaxedil

A. has no effect on the autonomic ganglia

B. causes bronchospasm from histamine release
C. both
D. neither   (3:394)

138. Leukopenia can be caused by

A. griseofulvin
B. urethan
C. both
D. neither   (3:512,591)

139. Alpha blocking agents are used in the treatment of

A. migraine headache
B. peripheral vascular disease
C. both
D. neither   (3:134)

140. Atropine causes

A. increased secretions of the pharynx
B. relaxation of the bronchial tubes
C. both
D. neither   (2:123)

141. Papaverine causes

A. constriction of the ureters
B. relaxation of the bladder
C. both
D. neither   (3:248)

142. Quinidine has

A. positive chronotropic action
B. negative inotropic action
C. both
D. neither   (3:150,151)

143. Thiazide diuretics

A. decrease reabsorption of sodium
B. increase reabsorption of potassium
C. both
D. neither   (3:207)

144. Thiazide diuretics potentiate

A. mercurial diuretics
B. antihypertensive drugs

C. both
D. neither   (3:207)

145. Side effects of procainamide include

A. hypotension
B. tachycardia
C. both
D. neither   (3:153)

146. Procaine is

A. a synthetic anesthetic
B. insoluble in water
C. both
D. neither   (3:315)

147. Luminal (phenobarbital) is used as a hypnotic in

A. chorea
B. gastrointestinal neuroses
C. both
D. neither   (3:275)

148. Bactericidal antibiotics include

A. erythromycin
B. tetracycline
C. both
D. neither   (3:567)

149. Penicillin is effective against

A. malaria
B. amebiasis
C. both
D. neither   (3:571)

150. The tetracyclines are active against

A. gram-negative bacteria
B. gram-positive bacteria
C. both
D. neither   (3:578)

151. Quinactine hydrochloride is used in the treatment of

A. malaria
B. trypanosomiasis
C. both
D. neither   (3:603)

152. Coumarin derivatives are useful in

A. recurrent phlebitis
B. hypertension
C. both
D. neither   (3:130)

153. Dehydrocholic acid increases

A. bile volume
B. total bile acid quantity
C. both
D. neither   (3:419)

154. The universal antidote contains

A. tannic acid
B. amyl nitrate
C. both
D. neither   (3:639)

Each statement is followed by four suggested answers. Answer according to the following key:

A. if answers 1, 2, and 3 are correct
B. if answers 1 and 3 are correct
C. if answers 2 and 4 are correct
D. if only 4 is correct
E. if all are correct

155. Medications applied to the skin may cause

1. vasoconstriction
2. inhibition of growth of microorganisms
3. soothing effect
4. removal of crust   (3:55)

156. Preparations of ephedrine include ephedrine sulfate

1. capsules
2. injection
3. solution
4. syrup   (3:110)

157. Papaverine has a relaxing effect on the

1. coronary arteries
2. bronchi
3. ureters
4. biliary system   (3:247)

158. Morphine is contraindicated in patients with

    1. bronchial asthma
    2. hypertrophy of the prostate
    3. stricture of the urethra
    4. renal colic   (3:244)

159. Morphine causes

    1. rise in the pain threshold
    2. stimulation of the cough center
    3. cortical sedation
    4. depression of the vomiting center   (3:248)

160. Morphine causes

    1. constipation
    2. pupil constriction
    3. depression of respiration
    4. decreased intrabiliary pressure (3:241)

161. Methadone

    1. is an opiate
    2. relieves cough
    3. does not cause drug dependence
    4. suppresses the cough reflex   (3:333)

162. The cough reflex is suppressed by

    1. morphine
    2. ipecac syrup
    3. dihydromorphinone
    4. terpin hydrate   (3:332)

163. Alkaloids of Rauwolfia are not recommended for patients with

    1. peptic ulcer
    2. colitis
    3. mental depression
    4. bronchial asthma   (3:162)

164. Side effects from the use of reserpine include

    1. nosebleeds
    2. constipation
    3. insomnia
    4. weight loss   (3:163)

165. Chloral hydrate is

    1. the oldest hypnotic
    2. a crystalline substance
    3. soluble in water
    4. insoluble in alcohol   (3:278)

166. Dilantin

    1. may cause gastric irritation
    2. is strongly alkaline in solution
    3. acts on the cerebral cortex
    4. is an anticonvulsant   (3:288)

167. Picrotoxin causes

    1. decreased respiration
    2. decreased blood pressure
    3. increased heart rate
    4. emesis   (3:239)

168. Symptoms of peripheral neuritis from isoniazid include

    1. numbness
    2. pain
    3. tingling
    4. inability to grasp objects   (3:598)

169. Caffeine causes

    1. decreased flow of urine
    2. decreased cardiac output
    3. decreased cardiac rate
    4. increased output of pepsin   (3:235)

170. Examples of diuretics that inhibit reabsorption of sodium include

    1. mercurials
    2. xanthines
    3. ethacrynic acid
    4. carbonic anhydrase inhibitors (3:202)

171. Inadequate response to diuretic therapy may be seen in cases of

    1. low output heart failure
    2. impaired lymphatic drainage
    3. cirrhosis
    4. nephrosis   (3:204)

172. Side effects of diuretic therapy include

    1. hypokalemia
    2. low serum uric acid
    3. impaired glucose tolerance
    4. hypernatremia   (3:204)

173. Toxic reactions to mercurial diuretics include

    1. albuminuria
    2. hematuria
    3. stomatitis
    4. hypertrophy of the gums   (3:206)

174. Spironolactone

    1. is administered parenterally
    2. is poorly absorbed from the gastrointestinal tract
    3. promotes the retention of sodium
    4. increases the retention of potassium   (3:211)

175. Prolonged use of mercurial diuretics increases the excretion of

    1. potassium
    2. calcium
    3. magnesium
    4. iron   (3:205)

176. Mannitol

    1. is a sugar alcohol
    2. is not reabsorbed by the tubules
    3. is an osmotic diuretic
    4. can be used to relieve cerebral edema   (3:213)

177. Symptoms of poisoning with salicylates include

    1. respiratory alkalosis
    2. hyperpnea
    3. metabolic acidosis
    4. hypoprothrombinemia   (3:629)

178. Symptoms of barbiturate poisoning include

    1. hypertension
    2. respiratory depression
    3. constriction of the pupils
    4. hypothermia   (3:629)

179. A patient suffering from glutethimide poisoning may require

    1. gastric lavage
    2. respiratory assistance
    3. renal dialysis
    4. diuresis   (3:629)

180. Continued use of amphetamine may cause

    1. anorexia
    2. irritability
    3. sleeplessness
    4. dizziness   (3:237)

181. Bacterial antibiotics include

    1. neomycin
    2. polymycin
    3. kanamycin
    4. chloramphenicol   (3:567)

182. Bacitracin is effective against

    1. streptococci
    2. pneumococci
    3. corynebacteria
    4. gram-negative bacteria   (3:591)

183. Griseofulvin can cause

    1. leukocytosis
    2. skin eruption
    3. constipation
    4. headache   (3:591)

184. Furadantin is active against

    1. viruses
    2. *Staphylococcus aureus*
    3. fungi
    4. *Escherichia coli*   (3:217)

Directions: Each group of numbered words and statements is followed by the same number of lettered words, phrases, or statements. For each numbered word or statement, choose the lettered item that is most closely related to it.

Questions 185 to 188

185. Sedative

186. Stimulant

187. Emetic A
188. Diuretic C

    A. Ipecac
    B. Phenobarbitol
    C. Caffeine
    D. Strychnine   (3:205,271,275,421)

Questions 189 to 192

D 189. The drug of choice in hookworm infection
A 190. A blood pressure reducing agent
C 191. A chemical congener of nitrogen mustard
B 192. A gel with high acid combining power

    A. Apresoline
    B. Aluminum hydroxide
    C. Thio-tepa
    D. Tetrachloroethylene
        (3:166,415,504,611)

Questions 193 to 197

D 193. Antergan
C 194. Decadron
B 195. Ipecac
A 196. Doriden
E 197. Tincture of opium

    A. Used as a mild hypnotic
    B. Used as an expectorant
    C. Bronchial asthma
    D. Urticaria
    E. Diarrhea   (3:225,246,277,334,470)

Questions 198 to 202

198. May cause hypertrophic gingivitis
199. A barbiturate
200. An ataractic drug useful in the management of obsessional states
201. May be used to relieve tremor in extrapyramidal lesions
202. A sedative that may be given to restless alcoholics

    A. Hydantoin
    B. Hyoscine hydrobromide
    C. Paraldehyde
    D. Pentothal
    E. Chlorpromazine
        (3:124,286,288,310,352)

Questions 203 to 206

203. Used as treatment for postoperative hiccup
204. A local anesthetic
205. Can relieve postoperative difficulty in micturition
206. A respiratory stimulant

    A. Cocaine
    B. Neostigmine
    C. Carbon dioxide
    D. Metrazol   (3:215,313,328)

Questions 207 to 234

Match the following drugs with the correct adult dosage

207. Morphine
208. Demerol
209. Codeine phosphate
210. Methergine maleate
211. Aminophylline

    A. 50 mg
    B. 100 mg
    C. 10 mg
    D. 0.5 g
    E. 0.2 mg   (3:205,246,249,526)

212. Atropine
213. Benadryl
214. Sparine
215. Chlor-Trimeton
216. Butazolidin

    A. 0.4 mg
    B. 0.5 g
    C. 30 mg
    D. 50 mg
    E. 4 mg   (3:123,224,225,262,359)

217. Nitroglycerin
218. Adrenalin
219. Luminal
220. Aspirin
221. Librium

    A. 1.0 mg
    B. 0.5 g
    C. 10 to 25 mg
    D. 0.4 mg
    E. 15 to 60 mg (3:105,157,259,272,360)

222. Trimethadione
223. Tigan
224. Serpasil
225. Chloral hydrate
226. Neostigmine

A. 300 mg
B. 2 mg
C. 1 to 2 mg
D. 0.2 mg
E. 0.1 mg   (3:128,163,227,279,290)

227. Glucagon
228. Compazine
229. Orinase
230. DBI

A. 1 mg
B. 1.0 g
C. 25 mg
D. 10 mg   (3:355,473,480)

231. Methadone
232. Nisentil
223. Pantopon
234. Dilaudid

A. 2 mg
B. 7.5 mg
C. 20 mg
D. 50 mg   (3:249)

Questions 235 to 250
Match the following drugs with the diseases they are used for

235. Cortisone
236. Dicumarol
237. Furadantin
238. Antabuse
239. Salicylates

A. Urinary tract infections
B. Allergic reactions
C. Alcoholism
D. Coronary thrombosis
E. Rheumatic fever
     (3:186,216,258,285,466)

240. Furadantin
241. Coly-Mycin
242. Chloroquine
243. Vioform
244. Flagyl

A. Malaria
B. Intestinal amebiasis
C. Bacterial enteritis
D. Urinary infections
E. Trichomonas vaginitis
     (3:216,592,603,607,613)

245. Iron
246. Sulfonamides
247. Streptomycin
248. Vasopressin
249. Cytoxan
250. Colchicine

A. Meningococcal meningitis
B. Tuberculosis
C. Hypochromic anemia
D. Diabetes insipidus
E. Leukemia
F. Gout   (3:175,455,505,561,581)

Answer Key: Pharmacology

1. A	33. E	65. B	97. C	129. D	161. C	193. D	225. B
2. C	34. A	66. A	98. C	130. C	162. B	194. C	226. D
3. B	35. A	67. A	99. C	131. C	163. A	195. B	227. A
4. D	36. E	68. C	100. B	132. A	164. B	196. A	228. D
5. E	37. B	69. C	101. C	133. B	165. A	197. E	229. B
6. C	38. E	70. C	102. A	134. A	166. E	198. A	230. C
7. A	39. A	71. A	103. B	135. A	167. D	199. D	231. B
8. D	40. B	72. C	104. C	136. B	168. E	200. E	232. D
9. E	41. D	73. C	105. B	137. A	169. D	201. B	233. C
10. D	42. C	74. A	106. D	138. C	170. E	202. C	234. A
11. C	43. E	75. D	107. A	139. C	171. E	203. C	235. B
12. A	44. A	76. A	108. A	140. B	172. B	204. A	236. D
13. A	45. C	77. D	109. B	141. B	173. A	205. B	237. A
14. D	46. D	78. B	110. A	142. B	174. C	206. D	238. C
15. D	47. A	79. C	111. C	143. A	175. A	207. C	239. E
16. C	48. C	80. D	112. A	144. C	176. E	208. B	240. D
17. A	49. B	81. C	113. C	145. C	177. E	209. A	241. C
18. E	50. A	82. B	114. D	146. A	178. C	210. E	242. A
19. A	51. A	83. C	115. A	147. C	179. E	211. D	243. B
20. A	52. A	84. C	116. B	148. D	180. E	212. A	244. E
21. E	53. D	85. C	117. C	149. D	181. A	213. C	245. C
22. E	54. A	86. B	118. C	150. C	182. A	214. D	246. A
23. E	55. E	87. A	119. B	151. A	183. C	215. E	247. B
24. C	56. B	88. D	120. D	152. A	184. C	216. B	248. D
25. C	57. C	89. C	121. C	153. A	185. B	217. D	249. E
26. C	58. C	90. C	122. C	154. A	186. D	218. A	250. F
27. D	59. C	91. C	123. C	155. E	187. A	219. E	
28. D	60. A	92. B	124. A	156. E	188. C	220. B	
29. C	61. C	93. A	125. B	157. E	189. D	221. C	
30. E	62. A	94. C	126. B	158. A	190. A	222. A	
31. A	63. D	95. B	127. A	159. B	191. C	223. C	
32. D	64. A	96. B	128. A	160. A	192. B	224. E	

Chapter Four

Chemistry and Physics

Directions: Select from among the lettered choices the one that most appropriately answers the question or completes the statement.

1. The number of known elements is

   A. 70
   B. 72
   C. 83
   D. 103
   E. 202   (4:151)

2. The atomic weight of nitrogen is

   A. 1
   B. 14
   C. 16
   D. 32   (5:33)

3. The color of sulfur is

   A. green
   B. black
   C. red
   D. yellow
   E. blue   (5:213)

4. The most abundant element is

   A. hydrogen
   B. oxygen
   C. iron
   D. calcium
   E. carbon   (5:91)

5. Ozone is a special form of oxygen made up of how many atoms of oxygen per molecule?

   A. 1
   B. 2
   C. 3
   D. 5
   E. 6   (5:94)

6. The lowest temperature at which a substance ignites is called

   A. temperature of combustion
   B. absolute temperature
   C. specific heat
   D. utilization heat
   E. kindling temperature   (5:97)

7. Oxygen has a valence of

   A. 2
   B. 3
   C. 4
   D. 6
   E. none of the above   (5:54)

8. The chemical symbol for phosphorus is

   A. Cu
   B. Cr
   C. Po
   D. P
   E. Pu   (5:205)

9. The chemical symbol for iron is

   A. Fm
   B. F
   C. Fe
   D. Ir
   E. I   (5:286)

10. The chemical symbol for potassium is

 A. K
 B. P
 C. Pt
 D. Po
 E. Pa (5:252)

11. The most abundant metal in the earth's crust is

 A. iron
 B. copper
 C. tin
 D. lead
 E. aluminum (5:266)

12. The most active halogen is

 A. chlorine
 B. bromine
 C. fluorine
 D. iodine
 E. osmium (5:182)

13. The atomic weight of calcium is

 A. 23
 B. 31
 C. 40
 D. 55 (5:33)

14. The atomic weight of potassium is

 A. 39
 B. 40
 C. 56
 D. 32 (5:33)

15. The atomic weight of carbon is

 A. 8
 B. 16
 C. 23
 D. 12
 E. 1.0 (5:33)

16. All of the following elements are metals *except*

 A. silver
 B. iron
 C. sulfur
 D. copper
 E. gold (5:38)

17. The atomic weight of sodium is

 A. 23
 B. 13
 C. 29
 D. 43
 E. 18 (5:33)

18. The sum of the atomic weights of the formula of a substance is called

 A. relative weight
 B. molecular weight
 C. mole
 D. equivalent weight
 E. valence (5:50)

19. The valence of a metal in the free state is

 A. 4
 B. 3
 C. 2
 D. zero (5:55)

20. The molecular weight of calcium carbonate ($CaCO_3$) is most nearly

 A. 40
 B. 48
 C. 12
 D. 100
 E. 117 (5:50)

21. In the periodic chart, elements with similar chemical properties are found together in vertical columns called

 A. triads
 B. groups
 C. octaves
 D. periodic series
 E. none of the above (5:34)

22. Hydrolysis is a reaction between a substance and

 A. a base
 B. an acid
 C. water
 D. a salt
 E. hydrocarbons (5:122)

23. A substance that changes color at a definite pH is called

    A. hydronium
    B. inhibitor
    C. ionic compound
    D. halogen
    E. indicator   (5:126)

24. An alloy containing mercury is called

    A. alum
    B. buffer
    C. amalgam
    D. chalcocite
    E. carnallite   (5:284)

25. The number of molecules in a mole is called

    A. atomic number
    B. periodic number
    C. Avogadro's number
    D. Lavoisier's number
    E. none of the above   (5:117)

26. All of the following are nonmetals *except*

    A. chlorine
    B. fluorine
    C. potassium
    D. phosphorus   (5:38)

27. The oxidation number of a free element is

    A. zero
    B. 1
    C. 2
    D. 3
    E. none of the above   (5:139)

28. Kaolin is

    A. sodium thiosulfate
    B. ferrous sulfate
    C. aluminum silicate
    D. calcium carbonate
    E. calcium oxide   (5:269)

29. Galvanizing is a process in which iron is coated with

    A. copper
    B. aluminum

C. lead
D. zinc
E. nickel   (5:283)

30. The formula of calcium phosphate is

    A. $Ca(PO_4)$
    B. $Ca_2(PO_4)_2$
    C. $Ca_3(PO_4)_2$
    D. $Ca_3(PO_4)_3$ (5:54)

31. Hard water may be softened by the addition of

    A. $NaCl$
    B. $CaSO_4$
    C. Na_2CO_3
    D. KOH
    E. $NaOH$ (5:262)

32. The empirical formula of methane is

    A. C_3H_8
    B. C_4H_{10}
    C. C_6H_6
    D. C_2H_5
    E. CH_4 (5:307)

33. The compound C_3H_8 is also called

    A. butane
    B. methane
    C. methyl
    D. propane
    E. bauxite   (5:307)

34. The element necessarily present in all organic compounds is

    A. carbon
    B. oxygen
    C. hydrogen
    D. silicon
    E. nitrogen   (5:306)

35. What is the formula of phorphoric pentoxide?

    A. PO_5
    B. P_5O
    C. P_5O_5
    D. P_2O_5 (5:54)

36. The pH of a neutral solution is

    A. 0
    B. 1
    C. 7
    D. 14
    E. more than 14 (5:123)

37. The pH of water is

    A. 0
    B. less than 5
    C. 7
    D. 14
    E. 1 (5:125)

Answer the questions in this group by following the directions below. Select

A. **if only A is correct**
B. **if only B is correct**
C. **if both A and B are correct**
D. **if both A and B are incorrect**

39. Properties of matter include

    A. heat stability
    B. light stability
    C. both
    D. neither (5:4)

40. Which of the following are properties of hydrogen?

    A. lack of odor
    B. lack of color
    C. both
    D. neither (5:101)

41. Metals are good conductors of

    A. heat
    B. electricity
    C. both
    D. neither (5:4)

42. Bromine is

    A. a metal
    B. liquid at ordinary temperatures
    C. both
    D. neither (5:187)

43. Nonmetals are

    A. solids at ordinary temperatures
    B. excellent conductors of heat
    C. both
    D. neither (5:5)

44. Bases

    A. are oxides or hydroxides of metals
    B. neutralize acids
    C. both
    D. neither (5:60)

Each statement is followed by four suggested answers. Answer according to the following key:

A. **if 1, 2, and 3 are correct**
B. **if 1 and 3 are correct**
C. **if 2 and 4 are correct**
D. **if only 4 is correct**
E. **if all are correct**

45. Univalent metal atoms are contained in

    1. NaBr
    2. CaF_2
    3. KCL
    4. $Ba(SO_4)$ (5:54)

46. Bivalent metal atoms are contained in

    1. $Ag(NO_3)$
    2. $AlCl_3$
    3. CH_4
    4. $Cu(NO_3)_2$ (5:54)

47. Trivalent metal atoms are contained in

    1. $Bi(NO_3)_3$
    2. $TiCl_4$
    3. $Fe(PO_4)$
    4. $Ba(SO_4)$ (5:54)

48. Tetravalent metal atoms are contained in

    1. $Ag(NO_3)$
    2. SiF_4
    3. CaF_2
    4. CH_4 (5:54)

49. Oxygen is

    1. a colorless gas
    2. an odorless gas
    3. a tasteless gas
    4. heavier than air   (5:94)

50. Mercury can combine with

    1. oxygen
    2. sulfur
    3. fluorine
    4. chlorine   (5:284)

Directions: Select from among the lettered choices the one that most appropriately answers the questions or completes the statement.

51. A quantity that requires a specification of magnitude is called

    A. scalar quantity
    B. vector
    C. component
    D. convection
    E. energy   (4:33)

52. An example of scalar quantity is

    A. time
    B. energy
    C. mass
    D. speed
    E. all of the above   (4:33)

53. An example of a vector quantity is

    A. velocity
    B. force
    C. acceleration
    D. momentum
    E. all of the above   (4:33)

54. Scalar quantities can be

    A. added
    B. subtracted
    C. multiplied
    D. divided
    E. all of the above   (4:33)

55. The acceleration due to gravity is

    A. 3 cm per second

    B. 32 cm per second
    C. 32 ft per second
    D. 32 ft per second per second
    E. none of the above   (4:82)

56. The quantum theory was introduced by

    A. Crookes
    B. Roentgen
    C. Max Planck
    D. Einstein
    E. Hertz   (4:461)

57. Which of the following is *not* a scalar quantity?

    A. distance
    B. temperature
    C. acceleration
    D. mass
    E. electrical charge   (4:33)

58. Equilibrium means

    A. balance
    B. convection
    C. displacement
    D. gravity
    E. acceleration   (4:46)

59. When a displacement takes place during a time interval, the ratio of the displacement divided by the time is called

    A. acceleration
    B. velocity
    C. average velocity
    D. speed
    E. rotary motion   (4:70)

60. Two concurrent forces produce a maximum result when they act

    A. east and east
    B. east and south
    C. east and west
    D. east and north
    E. north and south   (4:36)

61. When forces act on an object simultaneously at different points, the forces are said to be

    A. concurrent

B. nonconcurrent
C. rotational
D. gravitational
E. none of the above (4:50)

62. One inch equals how many centimeters?

A. 0.254
B. 2.54
C. 25.4
D. 1.24
E. 12.4 (4:10)

63. A man is five feet tall. His height in inches is

A. 40
B. 45
C. 50
D. 60
E. 70 (4:9)

64. Physical quantities specified by direction and magnitude are called

A. vectors
B. degrees
C. components
D. equilibrium forces
E. scalars (4:33)

65. The magnitude of velocity is called

A. acceleration
B. speed
C. average velocity
D. displacement
E. rotation (4:70)

66. Pressure can be measured in

A. centimeters
B. inches
C. pounds
D. pounds per centimeter
E. pounds per square inch (4:6)

67. The kilogram is a unit of

A. length
B. time
C. mass
D. acceleration
E. none of the above (4:4)

68. The length of time required for a single vibration is called

A. amplitude
B. period
C. frequency
D. buoyancy
E. elasticity (4:116)

69. The maximum displacememt of a vibration from the equilibrium position is called

A. velocity
B. amplitude
C. overtone
D. harmonic motion
E. inertia (4:116)

70. The velocity of sound is approximately how many feet per second?

A. 110
B. 310
C. 610
D. 1100
E. 11,000 (4:421)

71. The capacity of certain substances to pass directly from the solid to the gaseous state is called

A. evaporation
B. sublimation
C. utilization
D. fusion
E. convection (4:207)

72. Heat may be transferred from one region to another by

A. conduction
B. convection
C. radiation
D. all of the above
E. none of the above (4:194)

73. The hotness or coldness of a substance is measured in terms of

A. temperature
B. calorimetry
C. specific heat

D. joules
E. radiation   (4:174)

74. One hundred centigrade degrees corresponds to

A. 30°F
B. 62°F
C. 132°F
D. 200°F
E. 212°F   (4:175)

75. Directly related to the temperature of an object is the

A. average kinetic energy of the molecules
B. mass
C. density
D. weight
E. acceleration   (4:174)

76. The device used to measure temperature is called

A. thermometry
B. thermometer
C. calorimeter
D. calorimetry   (4:174)

77. The unit for measuring temperature is the

A. calorie
B. kilocalorie
C. BTU
D. degree   (4:174)

78. One kilocalorie is the heat required to change the temperature of one kilogram of pure water from

A. 0°C to 1°C
B. 5°C to 10°C
C. 10°C to 15°C
D. 14°C to 15°C
E. 24°C to 25°C   (4:175)

80. The freezing point of water is at

A. 12°F
B. 22°F
C. 32°F
D. 62°F
E. 132°F   (4:175)

81. The centigrade temperature corresponding to − 4° Fahrenheit is

A. 20°C
B. 10°C
C. − 5°C
D. − 20°C
E. − 100°C   (4:175)

82. The "large" calorie is equal to

A. 10 calories
B. 100 calories
C. 1000 calories
D. 50 calories
E. 500 calories   (4:195)

83. The amount of heat which must be added to change ice to water at 0°C is equal to

A. 40 cal/g
B. 80 cal/g
C. 150 cal/g
D. 540 cal/g
E. 960 cal/g   (4:201)

84. Water left in an uncovered dish will disappear by

A. sublimation
B. evaporation
C. boiling
D. condensation
E. crystallization   (4:204)

85. A lens thicker at the center than at the edges is called

A. concave
B. converging
C. diverging
D. plane
E. none of the above   (4:275)

86. A lens thinner at the center than at the edges is called

A. concave
B. converging
C. convex
D. diverging
E. none of the above   (4:275)

87. When a beam of sunlight is passed through a prism a band of color is produced which is called

    A. dispersion
    B. diffraction
    C. spectrum
    D. polarized light
    E. diopter (4:274)

88. Of the following, the best electrical conductor is

    A. wood
    B. glass
    C. paper
    D. wool
    E. iron (4:307)

89. An example of a ferromagnetic substance is

    A. nickel
    B. iron
    C. cobalt
    D. all of the above (4:382)

90. Electromagnetic induction was discovered by

    A. Edison
    B. Faraday
    C. De Broglie
    D. Joliot
    E. G.P. Thomson (4:145)

91. The amount of energy acquired by an electron accelerated through a difference of potential of one volt is called a/an

    A. electron volt
    B. alpha radiation
    C. kilowatt
    D. kilowatt hour
    E. international ampere (4:330)

92. Cathode rays are negatively charged electrical particles called

    A. electrons
    B. protons
    C. neutrons
    D. isotones
    E. deuterons (4:406)

93. Radioactivity was discovered by

    A. Becquerel
    B. Madame Curie
    C. Roentgen
    D. Bohr
    E. Rutherford (4:487)

95. A milliampere is

    A. 1/10 ampere
    B. 1/100 ampere
    C. 1/1000 ampere
    D. 1/10,000 ampere
    E. none of the above (4:345)

96. Neutrons carry

    A. positive electrical charge
    B. negative electrical charge
    C. positive and negative electrical charge
    D. no electrical charge (4:306)

97. The terms positive and negative electrical charge were first used by

    A. Benjamin Franklin
    B. Marie Curie
    C. Planck
    D. Ohm
    E. Kelvin (4:306)

98. The mass of an electron is about

    A. 3 times the mass of a proton
    B. 10 times the mass of a neutron
    C. $1/2$ the mass of a proton
    D. $1/100$ the mass of a neutron
    E. $1/1840$ the mass of a neutron (4:306)

99. Magnetism is the property of a substance to attract

    A. copper
    B. gold
    C. iron
    D. silver
    E. carbon (4:382)

100. The change from liquid to gas at a temperature below the boiling point is called

    A. sublimation
    B. vaporization
    C. condensation
    D. evaporation (3:204)

Answer Key: Chemistry and Physics

1. D	14. A	27. A	40. C	53. E	66. E	79. E	92. A
2. B	15. D	28. C	41. C	54. E	67. C	80. C	93. A
3. D	16. C	29. D	42. B	55. D	68. B	81. D	94. B
4. B	17. A	30. C	43. A	56. C	69. B	82. C	95. C
5. C	18. B	31. C	44. C	57. C	70. D	83. B	96. D
6. E	19. D	32. E	45. B	58. A	71. B	84. B	97. A
7. A	20. D	33. D	46. D	59. C	72. D	85. B	98. E
8. D	21. B	34. A	47. B	60. A	73. A	86. D	99. C
9. C	22. C	35. D	48. C	61. B	74. E	87. C	100. D
10. A	23. E	36. C	49. E	62. B	75. A	88. E	
11. E	24. C	37. C	50. E	63. D	76. B	89. D	
12. C	25. C	38. A	51. A	64. A	77. D	90. B	
13. C	26. C	39. C	52. E	65. B	78. D	91. A	

Chapter Five

Medical-Surgical Nursing

Directions: Select from among the lettered choices the one that most appropriately answers the question or completes the statement.

1. When an electrocardiogram is taken, the patient is usually

   A. lying on his left side
   B. lying on his stomach
   C. sitting
   D. standing
   E. curled up   (9:285)

2. The most common cardiac emergency is

   A. auricular fibrillation
   B. ventricular fibrillation
   C. sinus tachycardia
   D. acute myocardial infraction
   E. sinus bradycardia   (9:304)

3. Assume that a cardiac patient regularly assigned for home nursing care has been receiving digitalis orally. On one of the nurse's regular visits, she finds the patient's radial pulse rate is 58. Nursing orders do not give specific directions regarding pulse. In this situation, it would be most advisable for the nurse to

   A. give no direction to the patient regarding medication but watch his pulse rate more closely on future visits for changes
   B. advise the patient to stop taking medication and tell him that she will report the pulse rate immediately to his physician
   C. report immediately to the physician her observations as to pulse rate as well as regularity of pulse, patient's appetite, presence or absence of nausea
   D. teach the patient how to take his pulse and instruct him to take digitalis if his pulse rate goes above 60   (9:320,321)

4. A patient with congestive heart failure should be carefully watched for signs of

   A. fatigue
   B. uremia
   C. pulmonary edema
   D. heart block
   E. bleeding   (9:315)

5. Dyspnea of a patient with congestive heart failure is best relieved by placing the patient in which postion?

   A. a supine position
   B. an orthopneic position
   C. Trendelenburg position
   D. Fowler's position
   E. Sim's position   (9:315)

6. Paroxysmal atrial tachycardia may be terminated with

   A. digitalis
   B. eyeball pressure
   C. vasopressors
   D. all of the above
   E. none of the above   (9:311)

7. Improvement of atrial fibrillation may be effected by

   A. adrenalin

B. quinine

C. quinidine

D. Mercuhydrin

E. penicillin (9:312)

8. Right bundle branch block is invariably a sign of

A. heart disease

B. abnormal conduction through the right branch of the bundle of His

C. interauricular septal defect

D. right ventricular hypertrophy

E. embolism (9:308)

9. The characteristic electrocardiographic alteration in hyperkalemia is

A. elevation of the S-T segments

B. heart block

C. increase in the height of the T waves

D. a variety of ectopic rhythms

E. decrease in the height of the T waves (9:88)

10. Hemoptysis is common in

A. mitral stenosis

B. aortic insufficiency

C. patent ductus arteriosus

D. tetralogy of Fallot

E. gingivitis (9:295)

11. The most common cause of mitral stenosis is

A. typhoid fever

B. diphtheria

C. rheumatic fever

D. rheumatoid arthritis

E. gout (9:295)

12. The earliest symptom in a patient with mitral stenosis is

A. hemoptysis

B. chest pain

C. cough

D. fatigability

E. none of the above (9:295)

13. In the absence of cardiac enlargement or other symptoms, a blood pressure reading of 210/100 mm Hg would suggest a diagnosis of

A. anxiety

B. sclerosis of the aorta

C. hypertensive heart disease

D. essential hypertension

E. clinomania (9:297)

14. Spontaneous hemorrhage during anticoagulant therapy in a patient may be expected if the prothrombin level drops below

A. 1%

B. 5%

C. 10%

D. 20%

E. 25% (9:305)

15. In essential hypertension, there is

A. an increase in systolic pressure and a decrease in diastolic pressure

B. a decrease in systolic pressure and an increase in diastolic pressure

C. an increase in both systolic and diastolic pressure

D. a decrease in both systolic and diastolic pressure

E. none of the above (9:297)

16. The most common cause of death from subacute bacterial endocarditis is

A. cerebral embolism

B. pulmonary embolism

C. congestive heart failure

D. cardiac tamponade

E. rupture of the heart (9:293)

17. The most constant feature of subacute bacterial endocarditis is

A. anemia

B. chest pain

C. fever

D. weight loss

E. hepatomegaly (9:293)

18. The symptom which is most likely to accompany shock is

A. high blood pressure

B. abnormally high temperature
C. a fast pulse
D. a strong pulse
E. bleeding   (9:79)

19. The skin of a patient in shock will be

   A. flushed
   B. pallid and moist
   C. hot and dry
   D. normal
   E. scaly   (9:79)

20. The breathing of a patient in shock will be

   A. gasping
   B. shallow and rapid
   C. shallow and slow
   D. normal
   E. slow and deep   (9:79)

21. One step in the treatment of shock is to

   A. keep the patient warm
   B. apply ice packs
   C. give cold drinks
   D. remove all clothing
   E. walk the patient   (9:80)

Directions: This part of the test consists of a situation followed by a series of incomplete statements. Study the situation and select the best answer to complete each statement that follows.

Questions 22 to 44
Mr. Brown entered the hospital with chest pains and is diagnosed as having coronary disease.

22. The chest pain in coronary disease is due to

   A. anemia of the myocardium
   B. constriction of the coronary veins
   C. irritation of the cardiac nerves
   D. all of the above   (9:303)

23. A factor associated with increased risk for the development of coronary artery disease is

   A. smoking
   B. high blood pressure
   C. low vital capacity
   D. all of the above   (9:301)

24. The diagnosis of anginal syndrome is best made by

   A. taking a good history
   B. an electrocardigram
   C. fluoroscopy
   D. a physical examination   (9:303)

25. In the patient with angina pectoris, pain can be caused by

   A. lifting heavy objects
   B. climbing stairs
   C. running
   D. all of the above   (9:304)

26. If the patient with angina pectoris is obese, he requires a

   A. low fat diet
   B. low calorie diet
   C. low protien diet
   D. high carbohydrate diet   (9:304)

27. The patient with angina pectoris finds relief with

   A. digitalis
   B. morphine
   C. nitroglycerin
   D. epinephrine   (9:303)

28. The mortality rate for a first attack of acute myocardial infarction is

   A. 5%
   B. 10%
   C. 20%
   D. 45%   (9:304)

29. In myocardial infarction, there is

   A. necrosis of the heart muscle
   B. inflammation of the heart muscle
   C. narrowing of the coronary veins
   D. thickening of the endocardium   (9:304)

30. The highest incidence of ischemic heart disease occurs in

   A. women

B. young adults
C. men 40 years of age and older
D. children   (9:300)

31. The patient with coronary occlusion is expected to have all of the following symptoms *except*

A. low blood pressure
B. rapid pulse
C. cyanosis
D. clubbing of the fingers   (9:304)

32. The patient with coronary thrombosis may also have

A. dyspnea
B. substernal pain
C. clammy skin
D. all of the above   (9:304)

33. A useful procedure for the diagnosis of coronary occlusion is

A. an EKG
B. a complete blood count
C. transamination
D. all of the above   (9:304)

34. The patient with coronary thrombosis may develop elevated

A. serum cholesterol
B. serum transaminase
C. blood sedimentation rate
D. all of the above   (9:304)

35. An electrocardiogram done on a patient with coronary thrombosis indicates a condition of

A. the coronary veins
B. the capillaries
C. the heart muscle
D. all of the above   (9:304)

36. When the patient was admitted with coronary thrombosis, he was given morphine sulfate in order to

A. relieve pain
B. relieve the dyspnea
C. raise the blood pressure
D. increase expectoration   (9:305)

37. If oxygen is ordered for the patient with myocardial infarction, its purpose would be to

A. relieve cyanosis or dyspnea
B. relieve anxiety
C. prevent infection
D. prevent shock   (9:305)

38. To increase the possibility of further extension of the thrombus, the patient who has had a myocardial infarction is usually given a/an

A. anticoagulant
B. antibiotic
C. analgesic
D. diuretic   (9:305)

39. When an anticoagulant is given to a patient, which of the following procedures must be performed daily?

A. sedimentation rate
B. urinalysis
C. complete blood count
D. prothrombin time   (9:305)

40. The prothrombin time in patients receiving anticoagulants must be maintained at approximately

A. 5 sec
B. 10 sec
C. 30 sec
D. 50 sec   (9:305)

41. A patient receiving anticoagulants should be watched for

A. dyspnea
B. bleeding
C. hypotension
D. vomiting   (9:305)

42. A complication of acute myocardial infarction is

A. cardiac rupture
B. cardiac standstill
C. irreversible shock
D. all of the above   (9:305)

43. A complication of acute myocardiac infarction is

    A. pulmonary edema
    B. pulmonary embolism
    C. ventricular fibrillation
    D. all of the above   (9:305)

44. The convalescent period for most patients following a coronary occlusion is

    A. 5 days
    B. 2 weeks
    C. one month
    D. 2 to 3 months   (9:304)

Directions: Select from among the lettered choices the one that most appropriately answers the question or completes the statement.

45. The etiology of Raynaud's disease is

    A. inflammatory
    B. neoplastic
    C. functional
    D. thermal
    E. none of the above   (9:348)

46. Raynaud's disease is characterized by

    A. equal frequency of occurrence on both sexes
    B. gangrene involving the skin and the muscles
    C. asymmetrical distribution between the sexes
    D. pain aggravated by cold
    E. pain aggravated by heat   (9:348)

47. Aneurysm of the abdominal aorta is usually caused by

    A. syphilis
    B. Erdheim's medial necrosis
    C. arteriosclerosis
    D. trauma
    E. hypertension   (9:348)

48. Hemophilia is a blood disease affecting only

    A. children
    B. elderly people
    C. males
    D. females   (9:379)

49. Hemophilia is associated with a deficient

    A. number of red cells
    B. number of white cells
    C. blood clotting mechanism
    D. absorption of iron
    E. absorption of sodium   (9:379)

50. The most common site of bleeding in hemophilic children is the

    A. spleen
    B. liver
    C. intestine
    D. joints
    E. brain   (9:379)

51. One of the more widely used hematinics is

    A. ferrous sulfate
    B. atropine sulfate
    C. sodium phosphate
    D. methenamine   (9:374)

52. Patients with pernicious anemia usually have

    A. hypertension
    B. hyperglycemia
    C. hypoglycemia
    D. hypochlorhydria
    E. polyuria   (9:374)

53. Leukemia is a disease of the blood characterized by a

    A. moderate increase in the red blood cell count and decrease in the white cell count
    B. marked decrease in the red cell count and an increase in the white cell count
    C. marked increase in the hemoglobin content
    D. marked decrease in the white cell count   (9:377)

54. Of the following, the one which is *not* a respiratory disease is

    A. bronchitis
    B. pneumonia

C. nephritis
D. croup   (9:409)

55. Most respiratory tract infections are probably caused by

A. fungi
B. viruses
C. bacteria
D. spirochetes
E. protozoa   (9:488)

56. The cause of lung atelectasis may be

A. neurogenic reflex bronchospasm
B. swelling and obstructuon of the bronchial mucosa
C. bronchial obstruction by mucous plugs
D. poor posture that favors hypoventilation
E. all of the above   (9:183,184)

57. The first symptom of spontaneous pneumothorax is

A. a tightening of the chest with or without dyspnea
B. acute dyspnea
C. an anxious facial expression
D. restlessness and anxiety   (9:518)

58. Acute spontaneous pneumothorax in a young man unaffected by pleural effusion or dyspnea is best treated by

A. withdrawal of gas from the chest
B. artificial pneumothorax
C. bed rest
D. oxygen inhalation   (9:518)

59. A patient with an asthmatic attack should not be given

A. epinephrine
B. benadryl
C. potassium iodide
D. ether inhalation
E. morphine   (9:509)

60. Spontaneous pneumothorax without apparent associated lung disease is most often caused by

A. pulmonary tuberculosis

B. bullous emphysema
C. lung abcess
D. carcinoma of the lung
E. a pleural tumor   (9:518)

Directions: This part of the test consists of a situation followed by a series of incomplete statements. Study the situation and select the best answer to complete each statement that follows.

Questions 61 to 79

Mr. Howard is a 60-year-old man admitted to the hospital with a diagnosis of chronic obstructive pulmonary disease, producing obstruction to air flow.

61. Pulmonary disease includes

A. asthma
B. chronic bronchitis
C. pulmonary emphysema
D. all of the above   (9:502)

62. Asthma is caused by

A. an allergic tendency
B. pulmonary fibrosis
C. a virus
D. none of the above   (9:508)

63. Asthmatic attacks most often occur

A. in the morning
B. in the spring
C. at night
D. after lunch   (9:508)

64. Asthmatic attacks may be precipitated by

A. changes in humidity
B. smoke
C. physical exertion
D. all of the above   (9:508)

65. Status asthmaticus refers to

A. a chronic condition
B. an initial asthmatic attack
C. a continuous asthmatic attack
D. an asthmatic attack caused by humidity change   (9:508)

66. Most asthmatic attacks subside in about

    A. 10 minutes
    B. 30 minutes to 1 hour
    C. 2 hours
    D. 4 hours   (9:508)

67. Drugs used in the treatment of asthma include

    A. epinephrine
    B. ephrine sulfate
    C. aminophylline
    D. all of the above   (9:509)

68. A complication of bronchial asthma is

    A. pneumonia
    B. emphysema
    C. tuberculosis
    D. pulmonary embolism   (9:509)

69. Epinephrine is useful in the treatment of asthmatic attacks because it

    A. relaxes the smooth muscles in the respiratory tract
    B. accelerates the heart rate
    C. decreases the breathing capacity
    D. stimulates the smooth muscles of the bronchus   (9:509)

70. Helium is used with oxygen for the patient with an asthmatic attack because it

    A. is cheaper than oxygen
    B. is not flammable
    C. can be inhaled with less effort
    D. is odorless   (9:508)

71. Coughing is a symptom in patients with asthma. To lessen its severity and help loosen thick bronchial secretions, the doctor may order a

    A. detergent drug
    B. sedative expectorant
    C. narcotic
    D. barbiturate   (9:508)

72. An asthmatic patient with respiratory difficulty should assume an upright sitting position because

    A. it stimulates breathing
    B. the lungs can expand more fully
    C. the respiratory muscles will relax
    D. all of the above   (9:509)

73. Intermittent positive pressure breathing (IPPB) is often ordered for patients with chronic obstructive pulmonary disease. IPPB may be used for all of the following reasons *except*

    A. decrease arterial oxygen saturation
    B. increase alveolar ventilation
    C. administer mucolytic agents
    D. administer bronchodilators   (9:503)

74. The nurse can help the patient cough by

    A. using manual pressure on the front and back of his chest
    B. placing the patient in Fowler's position
    C. usimg manual pressure on the upper abdomen
    D. all of the above   (9:504)

75. Patients with chronic bronchitis have

    A. reduced vital capacity
    B. increased residual volume
    C. reduced expiratory flow rate
    D. all of the above   (9:502)

76. Patients with emphysema have

    A. decreased expiratory flow rate
    B. increased residual volume
    C. increased total lung capacity
    D. all of the above   (9:502)

77. In pulmonary emphysema,

    A. the lungs are not properly ventilated
    B. the po_2 may be decreased
    C. the pco_2 may be normal
    D. all of the above   (9:502)

78. Postural drainage is prescribed for the patient who

    A. is cyanotic
    B. has difficulty in raising sputum
    C. has increased residual volume
    D. cannot cough   (9:512)

79. The position assumed for postural drainage depends upon the

    A. weight of the patient
    B. age of the patient
    C. part of the lung affected
    D. type of medication taken before (9:513)

Questions 80 to 92

Mr. Johnson is a 40-year-old man admitted to the hospital with a diagnosis of pulmonary tuberculosis. The patient has a history of coughing with expectoration.

80. Nursing care includes all of the following *except*

    A. noting the color of the sputum
    B. noting the consistency of the sputum
    C. noting the volume of the sputum
    D. doing a culture of the sputum   (9:484)

81. Tuberculosis is usually transmitted by

    A. animals
    B. inhalation of droplets
    C. contaminated water
    D. contaminated milk   (9:495)

82. A positive diagnosis of pulmonary tuberculosis is made by

    A. sputum examination and x-ray examination
    B. blood count
    C. sedimentation rate
    D. gastric analysis   (9:496)

83. All of the following are tests for the diagnosis of pulmonary tuberculosis *except*

    A. Mantoux test
    B. Tine test
    C. BCG
    D. Sterneedle tuberculin test   (9:496)

84. Interpretation of the Mantoux test can be made after

    A. 6 hours
    B. 12 hours
    C. 48 hours
    D. one week   (9:496)

85. A positive tuberculin test indicates that

    A. infection has occurred
    B. the lung has necrotic tissue and caseation
    C. the patient has never been exposed to the tubercle bacillus
    D. an active infection exists   (9:496)

86. Tubercular lungs are characterized by

    A. scars
    B. nuclei
    C. tubercles
    D. ulcers   (9:495)

87. The causative organism of tuberculosis is

    A. gram-positive
    B. gram-negative
    C. similar to a virus
    D. able to grow in any media   (9:495)

88. Inhalation of mycobacterium causes inflammation in the

    A. pleura
    B. bronchi
    C. alveoli
    D. trachea   (9:495)

89. Drugs used in the treatment of pulmonary tuberculosis include

    A. PAS
    B. isoniazid
    C. streptomycin
    D. all of the above   (9:498)

90. Prophylactic treatment for pulmonary tuberculosis consists of

    A. bed rest for 3 months
    B. administration of isoniazid for one year
    C. administration of streptomycin for 6 months
    D. none of the above   (9:494)

91. Surgical treatment for pulmonary tuberculosis includes

    A. lobectomy
    B. pneumonectomy
    C. segmental lobe resection

D. all of the above (9:501)

92. Parts of the body subject to tuberculosis include the

A. larynx
B. skeletal system
C. nervous system
D. all of the above (9:501)

Directions: Select from among the lettered choices the one that most appropriately answers the question or completes the statement

93. The most common obstructive lesion of the esophagus is caused by

A. ingestion of lye
B. ingestion of hot liquids
C. carcinoma
D. benign tumors
E. none of the above (9:588)

94. Food poisoning is characterized by

A. abdominal cramps
B. explosive diarrhea
C. nausea
D. vomiting
E. all of the above (9:233)

95. In the case of food poisoning, of the following diets, the one which should generally be prescribed is

A. low-calorie fluid diet
B. high-calorie fluid diet
C. low-carbohydrate diet
D. low-purine diet (9:233)

96. All of the following are typical of gastric ulcer *except*

A. epigastric pain
B. eructation
C. relief of discomfort by alkalies
D. diarrhea (9:594)

97. A peptic ulcer is

A. more common in women
B. rarely cured

C. a lesion on the mucosa of the stomach or the duodenum
D. a lesion on the mucosa of the colon (9:593)

98. Most gastric ulcers of the stomach occur in the

A. lesser curvature
B. greater curvature
C. cardiac portion
D. pyloric region (9:594)

99. The "ulcer personality" possesses all of the following features *except*

A. perfectionism
B. agressiveness
C. excessive smoking
D. obesity (9:594)

100. A patient with a gastric ulcer should not be allowed to have

A. coffee
B. tobacco
C. tea
D. all of the above (9:594)

101. Drugs that can contribute to the development of peptic ulcer include

A. corticotropin
B. salicylates
C. phenylbutazone
D. all of the above (9:594)

102. The cause of peptic ulcer is

A. not known
B. poor eating habits
C. emotional personality
D. excessive use of alcohol (9:594)

103. The most characteristic complaint of patients with peptic ulcer is

A. epigastric pain
B. diarrhea
C. elevated temperature
D. painful defecation
E. none of the above (9:594)

104. An absence of free hydrochloric acid in the stomach of a patient with a previous history of peptic ulcer may indicate

    A. pyloric obstruction
    B. gastric malignancy
    C. gastric perforation
    D. all of the above   (9:582)

105. All of the following tests assist in the diagnosis of a peptic ulcer *except*

    A. stool examination
    B. urinalysis
    C. x-rays
    D. gastric analysis   (9:594)

106. Gastrointestinal series are useful in the diagnosis of peptic ulcer. This examination

    A. is the same as a barium enema
    B. is the same as gastroscopy
    C. requires the patient not to have food or fluids for 6 to 8 hours before examination
    D. does not involve x-rays   (9:579)

107. The purpose of a gastric analysis on a patient with peptic ulcer is to determine

    A. the presence of blood in the stomach
    B. the amount of free hydrochloric acid
    C. the presence of pus in the stomach
    D. all of the above   (9:582)

108. The drug used to stimulate the flow of gastric fluid during a gastric analysis is

    A. histamine
    B. atropine
    C. calcium carbonate
    D. sodium bicarbonate   (9:582)

109. In gastric analysis, how long does it usually take, after the administration of histamine, for the hydrochloric acid secretion to peak?

    A. 15 minutes
    B. 30 minutes
    C. 2 hours
    D. 6 hours   (9:582)

110. When histamine is given in a gastric analysis test, the stomach contents should be aspirated every

    A. 5 minutes
    B. 10 to 20 minutes
    C. 45 minutes
    D. 2 hours   (9:582)

111. Ulcer management includes

    A. restriction of alcohol
    B. use of antacids
    C. use of anticholinergics
    D. all of the above   (9:594)

112. Drugs used in the treatment of peptic ulcer will

    A. decrease gastric secretions
    B. lower the acidity of gastric fluid
    C. reduce gastric motility
    D. all of the above   (9:596)

113. Ulcer management consists of

    A. rest
    B. sedation
    C. bland diet
    D. all of the above   (9:594)

114. The diet for a patient with peptic ulcer usually consists of which of the following?

    A. frequent feedings
    B. small feedings
    C. non-irritating foods
    D. all of the above   (9:595)

115. Patients with peptic ulcers are often prescribed a

    A. Sippy diet
    B. low fat diet
    C. high carbohydrate diet
    D. Carrel diet   (9:595)

116. Milk, cream, and eggs are especially valuable in the treatment of peptic ulcers because they

    A. increase the secretion of hydrochloric acid
    B. are alkaline-forming

C. have laxative properties
D. lower the gastric acidity (9:595)

117. Concerning the diet used in the treatment of gastric ulcers, it is *not* true that

A. highly spiced food should be omitted
B. frequent feeding is usually ordered by the physician
C. milk and cream are usually the basis of the diet
D. citrus fruits are usually omitted because of their acidity resulting in a low vitamin C intake (9:595)

118. Patients with a peptic ulcer should avoid

A. gravies
B. meat soups
C. cola products
D. all of the above (9:595)

119. Complications of peptic ulcer include

A. pyloric obstruction
B. hemorrhage
C. malignant degeneration
D. all of the above (9:600,602)

120. The *least* common complication of duodenal ulcer is

A. intractability to medical care
B. common bile duct obstruction
C. obstruction
D. perforation (9:597,600)

121. Pyloric obstruction may be caused by edema of a peptic ulcer. A symptom of pyloric obstruction is

A. diarrhea
B. abdominal distention
C. projectile vomiting
D. thirst (9:600)

122. The symptom indicating perforation of a peptic ulcer is

A. diarrhaa
B. vomitimg
C. sudden severe pain
D. eructation (9:597)

123. The symptoms of a hemorrhaging peptic ulcer include

A. passing tarry stools
B. vomiting blood
C. drop of the blood pressure
D. all of the above (9:600)

124. If a patient does not respond to medical treatment, surgery may be indicated. Operations that may be performed include all of the following *except*

A. subtotal gastrectomy
B. total gastrectomy
C. vagotomy
D. colostomy (9:598,599)

125. Subtotal gastrectomy, sometimes performed on patients with peptic ulcer, involves

A. removal of one-half to two thirds of the stomach
B. closure of the duodenal stump
C. gastroenterostomy
D. all of the above (9:599)

126. The "dumping syndrome" sometimes occurs in patients who had

A. vagotomy
B. antrectomy
C. gastroenterostomy
D. all of the above (9:599)

127. The symptoms of the "dumping syndrome" can be minimized by

A. lying down after meals
B. drinking fluids with meals
C. eating foods rich in carbohydrates
D. all of the above (9:599)

128. The most common cause of death in patients with gastric ulcer is

A. bleeding
B. perforation
C. debilitation due to stenosis
D. malignant degeneration (9:597)

129. Acute amebic dysentery is most readily diagnosed by means of a

A. proctoscopy
B. stool culture
C. direct smear of the stool
D. complement fixation test   (9:610)

130. The first symptom of acute appendicitis is usually

A. nausea
B. diarrhea
C. constipation
D. periumbilical or epigastric pain (9:603)

131. A patient with acute appendicitis may have

A. fever
B. leukocytosis
C. nausea
D. all of the above   (9:604)

132. Acute mechanical intestinal obstruction may cause all of the following *except*

A. diarrhea
B. nausea
C. vomiting
D. distension
E. colicky pain   (9:617)

133. A male patient, age 45, is admitted to the hospital with the diagnosis of acute pancreatitus confirmed by physical and laboratory examinations. The presently accepted treatment immediately after admission is

A. immediate drainage of the pancreas
B. supportive intravenous therapy and bed rest
C. cholecystostomy
D. cholecystectomy   (9:654)

134. Patients with liver diseases should avoid

A. potatoes
B. white breads
C. alcoholic beverages
D. eggs   (9:639)

135. In a case where normal secretion of bile is prevented by disturbances of the liver or gallbladder, the dietician should recommend a

A. high fat diet
B. low fat diet
C. low purine diet
D. high calorie diet   (9:639)

136. The best diet in the treatment of diseases of the liver stresses

A. low protein, high fat
B. high protein, medium to low fat, high carbohydrate
C. low carbohydrate, high fat, high vitamin
D. high roughage, low protein, high vitamin   (9:639)

137. A patient with acute gallbladder is usually given a

A. low fat diet
B. 1000 mg sodium diet
C. high protein diet
D. low cholesterol diet   (9:655)

138. X-ray studies of the gallbladder are contraindicated in a patient with

A. fat intolerance
B. a food idiosyncrasy
C. iodine intolerance
D. a past history of hepatitus   (9:636)

139. Biliary colic is caused by

A. inflammation of the liver
B. inflammation of the gallbladder
C. obstruction of the bile duct
D. intrahepatic bleeding   (9:656)

140. Hepatocellular disease tends to decrease the serum level of

A. albumin
B. prothrombin
C. fibrinogen
D. all of the above   (9:633-634)

141. The disease characterized primarily by destruction of liver cells is

A. cystic fibrosis
B. cholelithiasis
C. pellagra

D. cirrhosis (9:646)

142. Liver function tests do not include

    A. glucose tolerance tests
    B. determination of alkaline phosphates
    C. determination of albumin-globulin ratio
    D. determination of serum sodium

    (9:634-35)

143. The purpose of a barium enema is to demonstrate

    A. the motility of the stomach
    B. any pathology of the bowel
    C. pathology of the stigmoid
    D. pathology of the duodenum (9:578)

144. The chief symptom of anal fistula is

    A. pain
    B. constipation
    C. fecal staining of the underclothing
    D. bleeding (9:629)

145. The most common symptom of cancer of the rectum is

    A. passage of red blood in the stool
    B. melena
    C. vomiting
    D. anorexia (9:625)

146. Diseases controllable by vaccination include

    A. smallpox
    B. tetanus
    C. yellow fever
    D. all of the above (9:273)

147. A method of active immunization now available is effective in the prevention of

    A. measles
    B. rabies
    C. poliomyelitis
    D. chickenpox (9:273)

148. An example of a contagious disease is

    A. the common cold
    B. hemophilia

C. appendicitis
D. glaucoma (9:489)

149. The gamma globulin fraction of pooled human plasma is an effective agent for preventing or modifying

    A. chickenpox
    B. measles
    C. scarlet fever
    D. diphtheria (9:275)

150. A disease transmitted largely through discharges from the mouth and nose is

    A. cholera
    B. dysentery
    C. hookworm disease
    D. tuberculosis (9:495)

151. The Frei test is used to diagnose

    A. pulmonary tuberculosis
    B. syphilis
    C. lymphogranuloma venereum
    D. gonorrhea (9:480)

152. The Mazzini test is used to diagnose

    A. syphilis
    B. leprosy
    C. tuberculosis
    D. malaria (9:475)

153. Hydrophobia is another name for

    A. tetanus
    B. infectious mononucleosis
    C. plague
    D. rabies (9:229)

154. Lockjaw is a synonym for

    A. measles
    B. tetanus
    C. hepatitus
    D. syphilis (9:60)

155. BCG vaccine is considered to give protection against

    A. smallpox
    B. tetanus

C. tuberculosis
D. tularemia   (9:495)

156. The disease which is generally considered to be caused by an infected wound is

A. bacillary dysentery
B. gonorrhea
C. malaria
D. tetanus   (9:60)

157. The cause of histoplasmosis is a

A. virus
B. fungus
C. parasite
D. spirochete   (9:515)

158. Erysipelas is commonly associated with infection by

A. *Staphylococcus aureus*
B. *H. influenzae*
C. *Escherichia coli*
D. *Streptococcus hemolyticus*   (9:713)

159. A presumed allergic reaction to streptococcal infection is

A. chancre
B. furuncle
C. variola
D. glomerulonephritis   (9:409)

160. An important factor in differentiating infectious hepatitis from serum hepatitis is

A. difference in incubation periods
B. degree of jaundice
C. presence or absence of gastrointestinal symptoms
D. characteristic abnormalities in hepatic function tests   (9:640)

161. The treatment of choice for infectious hepatitis is

A. choline
B. methionine
C. bed rest and diet
D. aureomycin   (9:643)

162. An example of viral disease is

A. trichinosis
B. relapsing fever
C. influenza
D. tetanus   (9:488)

163. All of the followimg are viral diseases *except*

A. yellow fever
B. mumps
C. influenza
D. actinomycosis   (9:711)

164. In acute gonorrhea, the diagnosis is verified by a

A. VDRL test
B. smear test
C. urinalysis
D. biopsy   (9:479)

165. Lymphogranuloma venereum is

A. also called climatic bubo
B. a viral disease
C. transmitted by venereal contact
D. all of the above   (9:480)

166. Syphilis is best treated with

A. sulphanilamide
B. gold
C. silver
D. antibiotic   (9:476)

167. The chancre in syphilis appears

A. approximately one year after infection
B. ten days to ten weeks after infection
C. within twenty-four hours after infection
D. three or four weeks after the appearance of the secondary stage   (9:475)

168. With reference to syphilis the

A. incubation period is 10 to 90 days with an average of 3 weeks
B. period of communicability is 2 weeks
C. mode of transmission is usually through indirect contact, as through towels and clothing

D. methods of control include routine taking of blood pressure (9:475)

169. The most effective and least toxic antibiotic used in treating syphilis is

A. streptomycin
B. aureomycin
C. penicillin
D. chloromycetin (9:476)

170. Penicillin is administered at regular and frequent intervals in the treatment of early syphilis because it

A. is important to keep the patient's temperature at a constant level
B. it is necessary to maintain the penicillin level in the blood at a determined concentration
C. encourages the patient to consume the desired quantities of fluids
D. keeps the patient from sleeping too long and sound, which is detrimental under these circumstances (9:476)

171. Syphilis is usually not considered contagious in the

A. primary stage
B. secondary stage
C. tertiary stage
D. chancre stage (9:476)

172. *Clostridium botulinum* may cause

A. meningitis
B. osteomyelitis
C. sinusitis
D. food poisoning (9:233)

173. The incubation period for botulism is usually

A. 3 hours
B. 10 hours
C. 15 to 24 hours
D. 2 days (9:233)

174. Botulism is a form of food poisoning usually caused by

A. the improper pasteurization of milk

B. disease carriers among food handlers
C. inadequate sterilization of preserved or canned foods
D. fungus growth in stale bread (9:233)

175. An effective drug for infections with acid-fast bacillus is

A. penicillin
B. streptomycin
C. erythromycin
D. aspirin (9:497)

176. The diet prescribed for the tubercular patient should contain at least

A. two quarts of milk daily, no matter what other foods are allowed
B. forced fluids containing at least 5000 calories daily
C. all of the foodstuffs in the normal diet with enough calories to maintain normal weight
D. a high vitamin C diet containing 5000 calories daily (9:500)

177. Of the following, the one capable of altering the course of tuberculosis is

A. streptomycin
B. BCG vaccine
C. the tuberculin test
D. the Schick test (9:497)

178. The most effective drug in the treatment of typhoid fever is

A. chloramphenicol
B. streptomycin
C. sulfaguanidine
D. aureomycin (9:611)

179. Acute glomerulonephritis is best treated by

A. rigid salt restriction and a high potassium diet
B. forcing fluids and restricting salt
C. rigid restriction and hypertonic salt
D. adequate fluids for turnover with adequate calories in the diet (9:409)

180. The nephrotic syndrome is a condition characterized by

A. edema
B. proteinuria
C. hypoalbuminuria
D. all of the above   (9:411)

181. Clinical characteristics of acute pyelonephritis include

    A. fever and pyuria
    B. bacteriuria
    C. pain in the flank
    D. all of the above   (9:408)

182. An inflammation of the pelvis of the kidney is called

    A. pyuria
    B. pyelitis
    C. pyemia
    D. pelvic inflammatory disease   (9:408)

Directions: This part of the test consists of a situation followed by a series of incomplete statements. Study the situation and select the best answer to complete each statement that follows.

Questions 183 to 198

Mrs. James was admitted to the hospital with the diagnosis of renal disease. The doctor ordered a P.S.P. test.

183. Concerning a P.S.P. test,

    A. it is used to determine renal function
    B. the dye is given IV
    C. fluids are given before the dye is injected
    D. all of the above   (9:387)

184. Renal function can be evaluated with

    A. blood chemistry tests
    B. urea clearance test
    C. urine concentration and dilution tests
    D. all of the above   (9:387,388)

185. Blood chemistry tests useful in evaluating renal function include

    A. blood urea nitrogen (BUN)
    B. nonprotein nitrogen (NPN)
    C. serum creatine level
    D. all of the above   (9:387)

186. An N.P.N. was ordered. The normal N.P.N. is

    A. 6 to 8 mg/100 ml
    B. 15 to 35 mg/100 ml
    C. 40 to 60 mg/100 ml
    D. 50 to 75 mg/100 ml   (9:387)

187. The ability of the kidneys to concentrate urine may be measured by

    A. the Fishberg concentration test
    B. the Addis concentration test
    C. the Mosenthal concentration test
    D. all of the above   (9:388)

188. Mrs. James was found to have an elevated BUN (blood urea nitrogen), possibly caused by a past attack of acute glomerulonephritis. Symptoms of acute glomerulonephritis include

    A. hypertension
    B. nausea
    C. headache
    D. all of the above   (9:409)

189. Symptoms of acute nephritis (Bright's disease) include

    A. hematuria
    B. decreased urine volume
    C. puffiness of the face
    D. all of the above   (9:409)

190. Laboratory findings in acute glomerulonephritis include

    A. high specific gravity of the urine
    B. casts in the urine
    C. albumin in the urine
    D. all of the above   (9:409)

191. Acute glomerulonephritis may be preceded by

    A. tonsillitis
    B. laryngitis
    C. sinusitis
    D. all of the above   (9:409)

192. The disease most likely to be followed by glomerularnephritis is

A. mumps
B. diphtheria
C. chickenpox
D. scarlet fever (9:409)

193. Symptoms of acute glomerulonephritis usually appear

A. 1 to 4 days after the infection
B. 1 to 4 weeks after the infection
C. 4 to 6 months after the infection
D. simultaneously with the infection (9:409)

194. All of the following are true about acute glomerulonephritis *except* it

A. is an inflammation of the nephrons
B. is usually seen in children and young adults
C. occurs more often in female patients
D. may follow an infection with scarlet fever (9:409)

195. Patients with acute glomerulonephritis require diets with reduced amounts of

A. protein
B. fat
C. carbohydrate
D. all of the above (9:409)

196. Patients with anuria resulting from acute glomerulonephritis require restriction of

A. fluids
B. potassium
C. protein
D. all of the above (9:409)

197. When caring for a patient with acute glomerulonephritis, the nurse should be alert for complications such as

A. cardiac failure
B. pulmonary edema
C. increased intracranial pressure
D. all of the above (9:409)

198. If the doctor wants x-rays of Mrs. James' kidneys, he will probably order

A. intravenous pyelogram
B. radiorenogram
C. cystogram
D. none of the above (9:388)

Directions: Select from among the lettered choices the one that most appropriately answers the question or completes the statement.

199. Treatment of acute cystitis includes

A. forced fluids
B. bed rest
C. sulfonamides
D. antispasmodics
E. all of the above (9:408)

200. Chronic cystitis may result from

A. prostatic hyperplasia
B. urethral stricture
C. inadequately treated acute cystitis
D. all of the above
E. none of the above (9:407)

201. Prostatic carcinoma usually metastasizes to

A. lung
B. liver
C. brain
D. bone (9:472)

202. The outstanding symptom in vaginitis is

A. fever
B. back pain
C. vaginal discharge
D. vaginal itching (9:451)

203. An excellent specific agent for the treatment of trichomonas vaginitis is

A. metronidazole
B. penicillin
C. erythromycin
D. sodium borate (9:452)

204. Pelvic inflammatory disease may be caused by

A. streptococci
B. staphylococci

C. *Mycobacterium tuberculosis*
D. all of the above   (9:454)

205. Chronic pelvic inflammatory disease is associated with

   A. pain
   B. sterility
   C. dysmenorrhea
   D. all of the above   (9:454)

206. Carcinoma of the vulva is usually associated with

   A. chancroid
   B. leukoplakia
   C. tuberculosis
   D. endometriosis   (9:463)

207. The most practical method for screening an asymptomatic woman for cervical cancer is

   A. cervical biopsy
   B. Papanicolaou smear
   C. culdoscopy
   D. curettage   (9:441)

208. The most frequent type of cancer in women involves the

   A. breast
   B. ovary
   C. tubes
   D. cervix   (9:734)

209. The most frequent ovarian tumors are

   A. fibromas
   B. carcinomas
   C. lymphomas
   D. cysts   (9:462)

210. "Chocolate" cysts of the ovary are associated with

   A. endometriosis
   B. pregnancy
   C. pelvic inflammatory disease
   D. none of the above   (9:463)

211. The most common site of breast carcinoma is

   A. above the nipple
   B. below the nipple
   C. upper outer quadrant
   D. upper inner quadrant   (9:735)

212. The most common and earliest recognizable sign of cancer of the breast is

   A. pain in the breast
   B. nipple discharge
   C. lump in the breast
   D. enlargement of the breast   (9:736)

213. Common goiter is chiefly due to

   A. an excess of carbohydrates
   B. a deficiency of iodine
   C. an excess of sodium chloride
   D. low basal metabolism   (9:666)

214. Of the following, the one *not* associated with hypoparathyroidism is

   A. muscle cramps
   B. high serum phosphorus
   C. cataracts
   D. renal calculi   (9:673)

Directions: This part of the test consists of a situation followed by a series of incomplete statements. Study the situation and select the best answer to complete each statement that follows.

Questions 215 to 240
Mrs. Brown, a middle-aged patient, was admitted to the hospital with a diagnosis of toxic goiter.

215. This condition is also called

   A. thyrotoxicosis
   B. exophthalmic goiter
   C. Graves' disease
   D. all of the above   (9:667)

216. In this condition, there is

   A. enlargement of the thyroid
   B. secretion of excessive quantity of thyroid hormone
   C. speeding up of metabolic processes
   D. all of the above   (9:667)

217. Hyperthyroidism is more common in

    A. men
    B. children
    C. older persons
    D. women   (9:667)

218. One of Mrs. Brown's chracteristic symptoms is

    A. nervousness
    B. lethargy
    C. anorexia
    D. vomiting   (9:667)

219. Mrs. Brown may also have

    A. tremor of the hands
    B. weight loss
    C. fatigue
    D. all of the above   (9:667)

220. Other syptoms of Graves' disease includes

    A. palpitations
    B. diarrhea
    C. increase in perspiration
    D. all of the above   (9:667)

221. Exophthalmos, a sign of hyperthyroidism, means

    A. poor vision
    B. double vision
    C. protrusion of the eyes
    D. myopia   (9:667)

222. The patient with hyperthyroidism requires all of the following *except*

    A. a high protein diet
    B. a high carbohydrate diet
    C. tea and coffee
    D. a high caloric diet   (9:669)

223. The doctor ordered a basal metabolism test for Mrs. Brown. This procedure requires the patient to be

    A. well rested
    B. calm
    C. awake
    D. all of the above   (9:665)

224. Patients given a basal metabolism test in the morning, must have

    A. nothing to eat after supper
    B. nothing to drink after supper
    C. 8 to 10 hours of sleep
    D. all of the above   (9:665)

225. Mrs. Brown is apt to have a basal metabolism of

    A. + 30
    B. 0
    C. − 10
    D. − 25   (9:667)

226. Treatment of hyperthyroidism by 1^{131} is contraindicated in

    A. pregnancy
    B. old patients
    C. thyrocardiac patients
    D. patients with recurrent exophthalmic goiter
    E. all of the above   (9:668)

227. Drugs used in the treatment of hyperthyroidism include

    A. propylthiouracil
    B. Lugol's solution
    C. radioactive iodine
    D. all of the above   (9:668)

228. Patients with hyperthyroidism are prescribed Lugol's solution because it

    A. reduces the metabolic rate
    B. reduces glandular vascularity
    C. helps prevent postoperative bleeding when a partial thyroidectomy is planned
    D. all of the above   (9:669)

229. Propythiouracil given to patients with hyperthyroidism

    A. interferes with the conversion of iodide to iodine
    B. causes atrophy of the thyroid
    C. causes hyperplasia of the thyroid
    D. promotes the utilization of iodine   (9:668)

230. Goitrogenic drugs are effective in the treatment of hyperthyroidism because they

   A. depress the pituitary secretion of thyrotropic hormone
   B. block the formation of thyroxine
   C. promote the absorption of iodine
   D. cause colloid to be deposited   (9:668)

231. Directly after a thyroidectomy, the patient is placed in

   A. Sim's position
   B. Fowler's position
   C. Trendelenburg position
   D. none of the above   (9:670)

232. Nursing care for a thyroidectomy patient includes

   A. protection of the suture line from strain
   B. help to raise secretions from the lungs
   C. observation for possible complications
   D. all of the above   (9:67)

233. Possible complications following thyroidectomy include

   A. recurrent laryngeal nerve injury
   B. tetany
   C. respiratory obstruction
   D. all of the above   (9:671)

234. Hoarseness associated with respiratory difficulty following thyroidectomy may be caused by

   A. edema about the vocal cords and the larynx
   B. hemorrhage
   C. injury to the recurrent laryngeal nerves
   D. all of the above   (9:671)

235. Respiratory difficulty (after thyroidectomy) caused by edema or nerve injury may require

   A. administration of carbon dioxide
   B. tracheotomy
   C. bronchoscopy
   D. administration of thyroxine   (9:671)

236. Complications following thyroidectomy may include

   A. tetany
   B. thyroid storm
   C. hemorrhage
   D. all of the above   (9:671)

237. If tetany complicates a thyroidectomy, treatment calls for

   A. thyroxin
   B. calcium
   C. magnesium
   D. cortisone   (9:671)

238. A patient with thyroid crisis may have

   A. hyperthermia
   B. increased pulse rate
   C. irritability
   D. all of the above   (9:672)

239. Treatment for thyroid crisis generally includes

   A. sedatives
   B. oxygen
   C. Lugol's solution
   D. all of the above   (9:672)

240. The cause of thyroid crisis is

   A. increased release of thyroxin in the circulation
   B. decreased production of thyroxin
   C. thrombosis of the thyroid artery
   D. none of the above   (9:672)

Questions 241 to 267

Mr. Smith, a 50-year-old man, has been admitted to the hospital with a diagnosis of diabetes.

241. Diabetes is

   A. more common in thin persons
   B. hereditary and transmitted as a mendelian recessive characteristic
   C. more common in men
   D. more common in persons under 20 years of age   (9:674)

242. Diabetes mellitus

   A. involves a disorder in carbohydrate metabolism

B. interferes with the function of the thyroid gland
C. interferes with the absorption of fats
D. all of the above   (9:674)

243. Diabetes is a metabolic disease characterized by

A. glycosuria
B. polyuria
C. hyperglycemia
D. all of ths above   (9:674)

244. Classic symptoms of patients with diabetes include increased

A. thirst
B. urinary output
C. appetite
D. all of the above   (9:674)

245. Mr. Smith was found to have hyperglycemia, a consequence of diabetes. Hyperglycemia means a/an

A. increase in blood sugar
B. decrease in blood sugar
C. decrease of sugar in urine
D. increase of sugar in urine   (9:674)

246. Mr. Smith's urine probably showed

A. hematuria, albuminuria
B. albuminria, pyuria
C. glycosuria, ketonuria
D. glycosuria, albuminuria   (9:674)

247. Mr. Smith's urine was examined with the Benedict test. When interpreting the results of the test, orange indicates

A. no sugar
B. 1 plus
C. 2 plus
D. 3 plus   (9:676)

248. Fractional urine specimens are collected from diabetic patients to determine

A. the amount of albumin in the urine
B. the amount of hemoglobin in the urine
C. the time of the day when excretion of sugar is heaviest

D. the amount of fat needed by the patient   (9:677)

249. Diabetics have difficulty with carbohydrate in metabolism due to insufficient

A. adrenalin
B. heparine
C. insulin
D. protein   (9:674)

250. Diabetic patients develop ketoacidosis which may result in coma when there is not sufficient insulin to metabolize glucose. The symptoms of diabetic coma include

A. drowsiness
B. nausea
C. fruity breath
D. all of the above   (9:689)

251. Diabetic coma may be precipitated by

A. infection
B. excessive food intake
C. failure to take prescribed insulin
D. all of the above   (9:689)

252. To treat diabetic coma, the doctor may

A. place the patient in oxygen tent
B. give insulin and IV fluids
C. order a high fat diet
D. order a low caloric diet   (9:689)

253. Since Mr. Smith uses insulin for his diabetes, he should know that insulin reaction may cause all of the following symptoms *except*

A. perspiration
B. increased thirst
C. hunger
D. tremor   (9:686)

254. Insulin reaction can also cause

A. irritability
B. weakness
C. blurring of vision
D. all of the above   (9:686)

255. A mild insulin reaction may be relieved by a

    A. piece of bread
    B. piece of fruit
    C. glass of orange juice
    D. piece of meat   (9:686)

256. The type of insulin that acts most rapidly is

    A. NPH
    B. regular
    C. protamine zinc
    D. globin zinc   (9:682)

257. The type of insulin that acts most slowly is

    A. ultralente
    B. lente
    C. crystalline zinc
    D. none of the above   (9:682)

258. The following insulin preparations appear yellow or cloudy *except*

    A. NPH
    B. lente
    C. protamine zinc
    D. regular   (9:681)

259. Insulin dosage is measured in

    A. units
    B. milligrams
    C. grams
    D. grains   (9:683)

260. Insulin is best administered

    A. intravenously
    B. subcutaneously
    C. orally
    D. intramuscularly   (9:682)

261. After administration, NPH insulin reaches its peak action in

    A. 2 to 4 hours
    B. 6 to 10 hours
    C. 8 to 12 hours
    D. 16 to 24 hours   (9:682)

262. Diabetics are prone to

    A. atherosclerosis
    B. retinopathy
    C. neuropathy
    D. all of the above   (9:691)

263. Orinase, an oral medication useful to some diabetics,

    A. lowers the blood sugar
    B. is an oral type of insulin
    C. comes in a liquid form
    D. all of the above   (9:685)

264. Orinase is effective in the treatment of

    A. juvenile diabetes
    B. severe diabetes
    C. diabetic acidosis
    D. none of the above   (9:685)

265. Nursing responsibility for a glucose tolerance test on Mr. Smith includes

    A. withholding food for 24 hours before the test
    B. withholding fluids for 24 hours before the test
    C. giving 40 units of regular insulin at the begining of the test
    D. none of the above   (9:677)

266. Mr. Smith's urine can be tested for sugar with

    A. Clinitest
    B. Tes-Tape
    C. Clinistix
    D. all of the above   (9:676)

267. The number of urine specimens collected in 24 hours for fractional urines is

    A. 6
    B. 5
    C. 4
    D. 2   (9:676)

Directions: Select from among the lettered choices the one that most appropriately answers the question or completes the statement.

268. Pathologic fractures may be caused by

    A. osteoporosis
    B. osteomyelitis
    C. tumors
    D. all of the above   (9:857)

269. After application of a splint to an extremity, which of the following conditions is an indication that circulation is impaired?

    A. elevated blood pressure
    B. lowered blood pressure
    C. tip of extremity is reddened and hot
    D. tip of extremity is blue and cold (9:859)

270. Rheumatoid arthritis

    A. attacks women more often
    B. is a systemic disease
    C. occurs most often in asthenic persons
    D. all of the above   (9:848)

271. The drug which has given new hope to victims of arthritis is

    A. ACTH
    B. histamine
    C. penicillin
    D. Chloromycetin   (9:841)

272. In the treatment of rheumatoid arthritis, cortisone

    A. may be routinely used
    B. cannot be dangerous
    C. should never be used
    D. may be beneficial in some cases (9:849)

273. A patient with uncomplicated acute rheumatic fever is receiving aspirin for symptomatic therapy. It is advisable to give this patient

    A. cortisone
    B. penicillin
    C. sulfaguanidine
    D. vitamin B₁   (9:853)

274. Gouty arthritis may affect the

    A. great toe
    B. ankles
    C. wrists and fingers
    D. all of ths above   (9:850)

275. Treatment for gout may include

    A. Probenecid
    B. colchicine
    C. salicylates
    D. all of the above   (9:851)

276. Benemid is useful in the treatment of gout because it

    A. decreases uric acid production
    B. decreases uric acid excretion
    C. increases uric acid excretion
    D. alleviates pain   (9:851)

277. Recurrence of acute gout is best prevented by regular administration of small doses of

    A. cinchopen
    B. colchicine
    C. salicylates
    D. Benemid   (9:851)

278. Broth is eliminated from the diet in gout because it contains

    A. an acid residue
    B. a high percentage of urea
    C. purine bodies
    D. too much vitamin B₁   (9:851)

279. Foods to be definitely restricted in a diet for gout are

    A. glandular organs
    B. sweets
    C. starches
    D. yellow vegetables   (9:851)

280. Tophi occur in

    A. osteomyelitis
    B. gout
    C. rheumatoid arthritis
    D. rheumatic fever   (9:851)

281. Subcutaneous modules are characteristic of

    A. gonorrheal arthritis
    B. osteoarthritis

C. rheumatic fever
D. tubercular arthritis   (9:852)

282. The most common type of eye disorder is

A. keratitis
B. conjuctivitis
C. hordeolum
D. refractive errors   (9:750)

283. Normal vision is represented by which of the following?

A. 20/200
B. 20/30
C. 20/20
D. 15/30   (9:752)

284. A vision defect is

A. aphasia
B. astigmatism
C. caries
D. toxemia   (9:750)

285. Of the following, the *least* accurate statement is that eyeglasses are prescribed in order to

A. cure infectious diseases of the eye
B. improve vision and relieve eyestrain
C. neutralize defects of focus of the eyes
D. strengthen weak eye muscles   (9:749)

286. Another term for farsightedness is

A. hyperopia
B. myopia
C. ophthalmia
D. astigmatism   (9:750)

287. The scientific term for nearsightedness is

A. hyperopia
B. astigmatism
C. myopia
D. emmetropia
E. glaucoma   (9:750)

288. Diplopia is

A. nearsightedness
B. farsightedness

C. double vision
D. spots before the eyes
E. normal vision   (9:763)

289. Retrolental fibroplasis is due to

A. exposure to high oxygen concentration
B. gonococcal infection
C. increased intraocular pressure
D. trauma   (9:768)

290. Strabismus is

A. the colored part of the eye
B. the middle coat of the eye
C. a deviation of one of the eyes due to a muscle defect
D. the white part of the eye   (9:763)

291. "Failure of muscle coordination to bring the image of an object upon the fovea centralis retinae at the same time in each eye" defines the condition known as

A. glaucoma
B. optic neuritis
C. retrobulbar neuritis
D. strabismus   (9:763)

292. A condition in which the lens of the eye becomes opaque is called

A. iritis
B. strabismus
C. cataract
D. blepharitis   (9:765)

293. Exophthalmos is often associated with

A. diabetes
B. hypothyroidism
C. hyperthyroidism
D. all of the above   (9:667)

294. "Pink eye" is a form of

A. keratitis
B. iritis
C. glaucoma
D. conjunctivitis   (9:761)

295. Night blindness is an early symptom of a deficiency of

A. vitamin C in the diet
B. vitamin A in the diet
C. roughage in the diet
D. thiamine chloride in the diet   (9:768)

296. Intraocular pressure can be measured with an instrument called the

A. opthalmoscope
B. oculometer
C. tonometer
D. mamometer   (9:752)

297. Determination of the intraocular pressure is important in diagnosing

A. astigmatism
B. myopia
C. glaucoma
D. conjunctivitis   (9:764)

298. A condition which in its advanced stage is characterized by symptoms of halos or rainbows around light is known as

A. cataract
B. detached retina
C. glaucoma
D. corneal ulcers   (9:765)

299. In uveitis, there is inflammation of the

A. external eye muscles
B. retina
C. iris
D. optic nerve   (9:763)

300. Drugs used for the treatment of glaucoma are usually

A. pupillary dilators
B. miotics
C. antibiotics
D. antiseptics   (9:764)

301. The term squint is synonymous with

A. strabismus
B. cataract
C. glaucoma
D. detached retina   (9:763)

302. The patient with uveitis complains of

A. photophobia
B. blurred vision
C. tearing
D. pain
E. all of the above   (9:763)

303. Keratitis means inflammation of the

A. iris
B. lens
C. eyelids
D. cornea
E. none of the above   (9:762)

304. Retrolental fibroplasia occurs in

A. premature infants
B. adults
C. young boys
D. diabetics
E. aged persons   (9:768)

305. In a cataract operation, the surgeon removes the

A. lens and its capsule
B. iris
C. iris and cornea
D. cornea
E. meibomian glands of the lids (9:766)

306. Otitis media is an inflammation of the

A. middle ear
B. inner ear
C. eardrum
D. mastoid
E. auditory nerve   (9:555)

307. The most common complication following a tonsillectomy is

A. cardiac arrest
B. hemorrhage
C. asphyxia
D. aspiration pneumonia   (9:543)

308. The main symptom of laryngitis is

A. cough
B. cyanosis
C. hoarseness
D. dyspnea   (9:544)

309. An important early sign of carcinoma of the larynx is

   A. chronic hoarseness
   B. regurgitation of fluids
   C. difficulty in swallowing
   D. respiratory distress   (9:551)

310. Pain of sciatica is usually aggravated by

   A. coughing
   B. sneezing
   C. defecation
   D. all of the above   (9:829)

311. A sudden onset of pain radiating down the back of the left leg with an absent ankle jerk in a previously well, 40-year-old man, suggests a diagnosis of

   A. lumbosacral sprain
   B. tabetic crisis
   C. herniated intervertebral disc
   D. silicosis   (9:829)

312. Features of compression of the spinal cord include

   A. motor weakness
   B. sphincter disturbances
   C. sensory objective disturbances below the lesion
   D. all of the above   (9:818)

313. A drug which has been used successfully in the treatment of epilepsy is

   A. Atabrine
   B. Sodium pentothal
   C. procaine oil
   D. Dilantin   (9:796)

314. A medication not used in the treatment of epilepsy is

   A. phenobarbital
   B. Dilantin
   C. neostigmine
   D. Tridione   (9:796)

315. Which of the following diets is the most effective in the treatment of epileptics?

   A. Sansum's basic menu

   B. ketogenic diet
   C. high protein menu
   D. low carbohydrate diet   (9:796)

316. Signs of viral encephalitis include

   A. fever
   B. drowsiness
   C. convulsions
   D. all of the above   (9:805)

317. Encephalitis lethargica is also called

   A. relapsing fever
   B. Bang's disease
   C. von Economo's disease
   D. Malta fever   (9:805)

318. Encephalitic manifestations may occur as complications of

   A. measles
   B. smallpox
   C. chickenpox
   D. all of the above   (9:805)

319. A drug that is used in the treatment of myasthenia gravis is

   A. curare
   B. neostigmine
   C. cortisone
   D. quinidine   (9:792)

320. Peripheral neuritis caused by isoniazid can be prevented if the drug is given together with

   A. pyridoxine
   B. folic acid
   C. thiamine
   D. insulin   (9:498)

321. Isoniazid neuritis is in part a manifestation of deficiency in

   A. pyridoxin
   B. thiamine
   C. vitamin B_{12}
   D. niacin   (9:498)

322. Parkinson's disease is marked by

   A. poverty of associated movements

B. postural changes
C. increase in rigidity
D. all of the above (9:791)

323. Parkinsonism is associated with

A. tremor
B. lesions of the basal ganglia
C. diffuse rigidity
D. all of the above (9:791)

324. A feature *not* usually associated with Parkinsonism is

A. tremor
B. diffuse rigidity
C. obsessional personality profile
D. intellectual deterioration (9:791)

325. An antibiotic producing a toxic effect on the auditory nerve is

A. chloromycetin
B. aureomycin
C. streptomycin
D. penicillin (9:560)

326. The cause of multiple sclerosis is

A. probably a virus
B. toxic substances
C. unknown
D. sodium deficiency (9:789)

327. The most common neurological disorder in which unwanted movements occur is

A. Parkinsonism
B. myasthenia gravis
C. diabetic neuritis
D. chronic mercury poisoning (9:791)

328. The drug of choice for migraine is

A. calcium lactate
B. histamine
C. Demerol
D. erbotamine tartrate (9:794)

329. A slowly progressive, degenerative disease of the nervous system usually occurring during or after middle life, characterized

by tremors and rigidity of the skeletal muscles, best defines the condition known as

A. arthritis
B. Parkinson's disease
C. Jacksonian epilepsy
D. multiple sclerosis (9:791)

330. A furuncle may arise from the penetration of a virulent staphylococcus through

A. a hair follicle
B. a sebaceous gland
C. a sweat gland
D. all of the above (9:712)

331. Erysipelas is commonly associated with infection by

A. *Staphylococcus aureus*
B. *H. influenzae*
C. *Escherichia coli*
D. *Streptococcus hemolyticus* (9:713)

332. Herpes zoster is related to

A. measles
B. mumps
C. chickenpox
D. scarlet fever (9:714)

333. The eruptions of herpes zoster most often occur in the

A. genital area
B. neck
C. thoracic region
D. cornea
E. soft palate (9:714)

334. An impact that produces interstitial hemorrhage without disruption of the skin is called

A. concussion
B. contusion
C. incision
D. laceration (9:59)

335. A vesicle is a skin lesion containing

A. pus
B. serous fluid

C. blood

D. serosanguinous fluid   (9:709)

336. Increased pigmentation of the skin can be caused by

A. hyperfunction of the adrenal medulla
B. hyperfunction of the thymus
C. hypofunction of the adrenal cortex
D. hyperfunction of the thyroid   (9:693)

337. Tinea of the scalp

A. is correctly called ringworm of the scalp
B. is a disease of children
C. may be treated with griseofulvin
D. all of the above   (9:710)

338. The causative organism of ''athlete's foot'' is a

A. bacterium
B. fungus
C. protozoan
D. roundworm   (9:711)

339. Ringworm is caused by a

A. bacterium
B. fungus
C. protozoan
D. roundworm   (9:711)

340. Impetigo contagiosa is a skin disease

A. caused by the itch mite
B. characterized by a scaly patch area starting at the hairline
C. characterized by a spotty rash commonly found on the covered surfaces of the body
D. characterized by vesicles, pustules, and crusts commonly found on the face and hands   (9:713)

341. Erysipelas most commonly involves the

A. face
B. neck
C. chest
D. thigh   (9:713)

342. A skin disease *not* caused by bacteria is

A. erysipelas
B. furuncles
C. carbuncles
D. ringworm of the scalp   (9:711)

343. Exposure to poison sumac is a common cause of

A. seborrheic dermatitis
B. psoriasis
C. erysipelas
D. allergic contact dermatitis   (9:74)

344. Of the following, the primary cause of acne in adolescents is

A. too much carbohydrate in the diet
B. the inability of the fat gland ducts and outlets to allow passage of increased secretions of sebum
C. lack of vitamin A in the diet
D. lack of good personal hygiene (9:712)

345. A possibly life-saving product in severe acute urticuria is

A. nicotinyl alcohol
B. atropine
C. Imuran
D. epinephrine   (9:715)

346. The best treatment for dermatomyositis is to administer

A. steroid drugs
B. edathamil calcium-disodium
C. testosterone
D. salts of para-aminobenzoic acid (9:8;4)

347. Pemphigus usually responds well to treatment with

A. penicillin
B. corticosteroids
C. hydroquinone
D. vitamin A   (9:711)

348. The drug of choice in tinea capitis is

A. vitamin A
B. trichloroacetic acid

C. cortisone
D. griseofulvin   (9:711)

349. Isonicotinic acid hydrazide is used chiefly in the treatment of

A. rheumatic fever
B. arthritis
C. cancer
D. tuberculosis   (9:497)

350. An overdose of heparin can be counteracted with

A. folic acid
B. lactone
C. protamine
D. whole blood   (9:342)

351. An overdose of insulin is likely to produce

A. nervousness, excessive hunger, weakness, and sweating
B. vomiting, labored respiration, and anorexia
C. polyuria, restlessness, and anhydremia
D. nausea, labored respiration, and dyspnea   (9:686)

352. A disease requiring restriction of fluids and salt is

A. acute nephritis with edema
B. anemia
C. pellagra
D. peptic ulcer   (9:409)

353. The usual duration of action of an intravenous dose of heparin is

A. ten minutes
B. half hour
C. one hour
D. two to four hours   (9:341)

354. The addition of fluorine to drinking water with a low fluorine level has the primary effect of

A. strengthening bones
B. improving skin texture
C. preventing dental caries
D. preventing scurvy   (9:567)

355. The glucose tolerance test diagnoses

A. ulcers
B. hypertension
C. leukemia
D. diabetes   (9:677)

356. A rising titer of heterophile antibodies is most characteristic of

A. infectious mononucleosis
B. dengue fever
C. measles
D. rheumatoid arthritis
E. mumps   (9:380)

357. Clinitest is used to test urine for

A. bile pigments
B. urea
C. acetone
D. sugar   (9:676)

358. The galactose tolerance test determines disturbances in

A. kidney function
B. gallbladder function
C. liver function
D. adrenal function   (9:634)

369. The Benedict test is commonly used to test urine for

A. sugar
B. acetone
C. blood
D. pus   (9:676)

360. A patient complaining of polyuria, extreme thirst, excessive hunger, loss of strength, loss of weight, and whose urine is of high specific gravity, is likely to have

A. diabetes mellitus
B. sprue
C. hyperthyroidism
D. nephritis   (9:674)

361. Interpretation of tuberculin tests is made after

A. 12 hours
B. 18 hours

C. 36 hours

D. 48 hours   (9:496)

362. Of the following drugs, the one that has been found useful in the detection of pheochromocytoma is

A. hydrazinophthalazine

B. Benzedrine

C. pyribenzamine

D. benzodioxane   (9:695)

363. Of the following conditions, the one which may be infectious is

A. hiatal hernia

B. angina pectoris

C. gonorrhea

D. leukemia   (9:479)

364. Salpingitis is an inflammation of the

A. ovary

B. cervix

C. Fallopian tube

D. vagina   (9:454)

365. The "dumping syndrome" occurs following

A. gastrectomy

B. splenectomy

C. herniorrhaphy

D. colectomy   (9:599)

366. An acid-fast bacillus is the cause of

A. tuberculosis

B. scarlet fever

C. diphtheria

D. mumps   (9:497)

367. Cholecystitis is an inflammatory condition of the

A. colon

B. kidney

C. bile duct

D. gallbladder   (9:655)

368. Cataract is a disease of the

A. ear

B. eye

C. lungs

D. liver   (9:765)

369. "Petit mal" is a form of

A. epilepsy

B. syphilis

C. diabetes

D. malaria   (9:795)

370. The term hordeolum means

A. chalazion

B. sty

C. ectropion

D. tinnitus   (9:761)

371. Of the following, the one that is *not* a collagen disease is

A. Hodgkin's disease

B. lupus erythematosus disseminatus

C. dermatomyositis

D. scleroderma   (9:377)

Answer the questions in this group by following the directions below. Select

A. **if only A is correct**

B. **if only B is correct**

C. **if both A and B are correct**

D. **if both A and B are incorrect**

372. Rheumatic heart disease is a complication of

A. rheumatic fever

B. rheumatoid arthritis

C. both

D. neither   (9:293)

373. Pericarditis is associated with

A. precordial pain

B. dyspnea

C. both

D. neither   (9:292)

374. Edema patients with heart failure can be controlled

A. by restriction of salt intake

B. with diuretic drugs

C. both
D. neither   (9:318,321)

375. Drugs used in the treatment of hypertension include

A. Aldomet
B. chlorothiazide
C. both
D. neither   (9:298-99)

376. Digitalis should *not* be administered to a patient who

A. has nausea and is vomiting
B. complains of headache
C. both
D. neither   (9:321)

377. A patient with congestive heart failure may have

A. pedal edema
B. dyspnea
C. both
D. neither   (9:314)

378. Symptoms which indicate left-sided heart failure are

A. ascites and anxiety
B. dyspnea and frothy sputum
C. both
D. neither   (9:315)

379. Symptoms of left-sided heart failure (secondary to coronary artery disease) are

A. dyspnea on exertion
B. paroxysmal nocturnal dyspnea
C. both
D. neither   (9:315)

380. The venous pressure is elevated in

A. congestive heart failure
B. constrictive pericarditis
C. both
D. neither   (9:286)

381. The venous pressure is elevated in

A. patients receiving digitalis
B. congestive heart failure
C. both
D. neither   (9:286)

382. Fallot's tetralogy comprises

A. dextrocardia
B. a septal defect
C. both
D. neither   (9:291)

383. Peripheral vascular diseases include

A. Buerger's disease
B. Raynaud's disease
C. both
D. neither   (9:347-48)

384. Thrombophlebitis

A. is the occlusion and inflammation of a vein
B. may result from early ambulation after surgery
C. both
D. neither   (9:353)

385. Raynaud's disease

A. does not improve with sympathectomy
B. usually first affects the tips of the fingers and toes
C. both
D. neither   (9:348)

386. Arteriovenous fistulas

A. may be congenital
B. can be caused by trauma
C. both
D. neither   (9:352)

387. Anemia may result from

A. blood loss
B. impaired production of blood cells in the body
C. both
D. neither   (9:373-74)

388. Sickle cell anemia is

A. a hemolytic anemia
B. characterized by the presence of an abnormal hemoglobin
C. both
D. neither   (9:376)

389. Polycythemia vera is associated with

A. an increased number of red blood cells
B. a decreased number of white blood cells
C. both
D. neither   (9:379)

390. In polycythemia vera

A. the higher number of red blood cells can cause embolic epidoses
B. radioactive phosphorus can be used as a therapeutic agent
C. both
D. neither   (9:379)

391. Hemophilia can be cured with injections of

A. iron
B. nicotinic acid
C. both
D. neither   (9:379)

392. Treatment of hemophilia includes

A. avoidance of injury
B. transfusions of fresh blood
C. both
D. neither   (9:379)

393. Hodgkin's disease

A. produces painless enlargement of the lymph nodes
B. responds to treatment with penicillin
C. both
D. neither   (9:378)

394. The treatment of Hodgkin's disease includes

A. x-ray therapy
B. nitrogen mustard
C. both
D. neither   (9:378)

395. Agents effective in acute leukemia include

A. Myleran
B. urethane
C. both
D. neither   (9:377)

396. The majority of patients with pneumococcal pneumonia develop

A. coughing
B. pleuritic pain
C. both
D. neither   (9:491)

397. A patient with bacterial pneumonia will exhibit

A. rapid breath sounds
B. fever
C. both
D. neither   (9:491)

398. Chronic obstructive emphysema is associated with

A. increased airway resistance
B. increased diffusion capacity
C. both
D. neither   (9:502)

399. Bronchial asthma is

A. a form or allergy
B. contagious
C. both
D. neither   (9:508)

400. Pneumothorax

A. refers to the presence of air in the pleura
B. may occur spontaneously as a result of lung disease
C. both
D. neither   (9:518)

401. In pneumothorax the

A. intrapleural pressure becomes equal to that of the atmosphere
B. lung collapses
C. both
D. neither   (9:518)

402. Acute pulmonary edema is

    A. a medical emergency
    B. associated with dyspnea
    C. both
    D. neither   (9:315)

403. Bronchogenic carcinoma

    A. is the most common type of lung cancer
    B. arises from the pleural epthelium
    C. both
    D. neither   (9:517)

404. Food poisoning can be caused by

    A. Salmonella organisms
    B. staphylococcus organisms
    C. both
    D. neither   (9:232,233)

405. A frequent discomfort of peptic ulcer is

    A. diarrhea
    B. eructation
    C. both
    D. neither   (9:594)

406. Symptoms of perforated gastric ulcer include

    A. shock
    B. abdominal rigidity
    C. both
    D. neither   (9:597)

407. Acute appendicitis

    A. occurs in both sexes
    B. requires surgical intervention
    C. both
    D. neither   (9:603,604)

408. Intestinal obstruction may occur in

    A. celiac disease
    B. abdominal hernia
    C. both
    D. neither   (9:617)

409. Symptoms of intestinal obstruction include

    A. vomiting
    B. obstipation
    C. both
    D. neither   (9:617)

410. Carcinoma of the colon may occur as a complication of

    A. multiple familial polyposis
    B. prolonged chronic ulcerative colitis
    C. both
    D. neither   (9:606,613)

411. Frequent passage of liquid hemorrhagic stools in patients with ulcerative colitis may cause

    A. hyperproteinemia
    B. iron deficiency anemia
    C. both
    D. neither   (9:606)

412. Rectal bleeding may be a symptom of

    A. hemorrhoids
    B. carcinoma of the rectum
    C. both
    D. neither   (9:625,627)

413. A fissure *in ano* concerns

    A. the anal mucosa
    B. the anal muscle
    C. both
    D. neither   (9:628)

414. Liver function tests include the

    A. van den Bergh test
    B. bromsulfalein test
    C. both
    D. neither   (9:633,635)

415. Complete obstruction of the common bile duct causes

    A. elevation of the serum bilirubin
    B. elevation of the serum alkaline phosphatase
    C. both
    D. neither   (9:635,638)

416. Immunization has resulted in a marked decrease in the incidence of

    A. infectious hepatitis
    B. tetanus
    C. both
    D. neither   (9:273)

417. Infections caused by streptococcus include

    A. erysipelas
    B. impetigo
    C. both
    D. neither   (9:713)

418. Infectious mononucleosis is characterized by

    A. lymphadenopathy
    B. absolute lymphocytosis
    C. both
    D. neither   (9:380)

419. Tetanus is

    A. caused by gram-positive rods
    B. also called "lockjaw"
    C. both
    D. neither   (9:360)

420. Patients with infectious hepatitis require a

    A. low protein diet
    B. low carbohydrate diet
    C. both
    D. neither   (9:644)

421. Gonorrhea

    A. is a venereal disease
    B. produces an ulceration on the external genitalia
    C. both
    D. neither   (9:479)

422. Chancroid

    A. is a venereal disease
    B. affects only men
    C. both
    D. neither   (9:480)

423. Chancroid is

    A. the initial lesion of syphilis
    B. caused by the Bordet-Gengou bacillus
    C. both
    D. neither   (9:480)

424. Lymphogranuloma inguinale is

    A. a venereal disease
    B. increasing in frequency all over the world
    C. both
    D. neither   (9:480)

425. Complications of lymphogranuloma venereum include

    A. rectal fistulas
    B. lymphedema of the legs
    C. both
    D. neither   (9:480)

426. Manifestations of late syphilis include

    A. syphilitic chancres
    B. condylomas
    C. both
    D. neither   (9:476)

427. Common infections transmitted by food include

    A. amebiasis
    B. Q fever
    C. both
    D. neither   (9:610)

428. A patient with acute nephritis should have

    A. restricted sodium intake
    B. increased potassium intake
    C. both
    D. neither   (9:409)

429. Acute cystitis causes

    A. dysuria
    B. urinary frequency
    C. both
    D. neither   (9:407)

430. Carcinoma of the prostate

    A. causes more deaths than carcinoma of the stomach
    B. usually arises in the posterior periphery of the gland
    C. both
    D. neither   (9:472)

431. Amenorrhea is a normal state during

    A. pregnancy
    B. lactation
    C. both
    D. neither   (9:451)

432. Secondary amenorrhea can be caused by

    A. organic disease
    B. endocrine disturbances
    C. both
    D. neither   (9:451)

433. Dysfunctional bleeding is synonymous with

    A. functional bleeding
    B. anovulatory bleeding
    C. both
    D. neither   (9:451)

434. The definition of menorrhagia describes cyclic bleeding which is

    A. prolonged
    B. excessive
    C. both
    D. neither   (9:451)

435. Menorrhagia is frequently caused by

    A. pregnancy
    B. uterine fibromas
    C. both
    D. neither   (9:451)

436. Menorrhagia is often the first symptom of

    A. thrombocytopenia
    B. salpingitis
    C. both
    D. neither   (9:451)

437. Menorrhagia may be caused by

    A. tumors
    B. functional factors
    C. both
    D. neither   (9:451)

438. Accepted treatment for acute bartholinitis includes

    A. douches
    B. antibiotics
    C. both
    D. neither   (9:453)

439. Flagyl is effective in vaginitis caused by

    A. trichomonas
    B. gonococcus
    C. both
    D. neither   (9:452)

440. Local estrogenic therapy is the treatment of choice for

    A. gonorrheal vaginitis
    B. senile vaginitis
    C. both
    D. neither   (9:452)

441. Endometriosis can cause

    A. dysmenorrhea
    B. dyspareunia
    C. both
    D. neither   (9:463)

442. Pelvic inflammatory disease may include the

    A. ovaries
    B. fallopian tubes
    C. both
    D. neither   (9:453)

443. Endometriosis can be successfully treated with

    A. cortisone
    B. progesterone
    C. both
    D. neither   (9:463)

444. Uterine myomas are caused by

A. pregnancy
B. abnormal ovarian function
C. both
D. neither   (9:462)

445. Basic metabolic rate

A. measures the amount of oxygen used at rest
B. is low in hyperthyroidism
C. both
D. neither   (9:665)

446. Hyperthyroidism is often associated with

A. exophthalmos
B. low basal metabolic rate
C. both
D. neither   (9:667)

447. Hyperfunction of the thyroid gland causes

A. decreased appetite
B. somnolence
C. both
D. neither   (9:667)

448. In hyperthyroidism the

A. blood serum cholesterol is decreased
B. patient has a feeling of fatigue
C. both
D. neither   (9:666,667)

449. Thyroid crisis

A. is usually precipitated by surgery
B. manifests itself by rapid pulse and restlessness
C. both
D. neither   (9:671-72)

450. Hyperparathyroidism

A. causes tetany
B. is characterized by low blood calcium
C. both
D. neither   (9:673)

451. Hyperparathyroidism

A. may result from a parathyroid tumor
B. leads to increased excretion of calcium in the urine

C. both
D. neither   (9:673)

452. Patients with diabetes insipidus

A. excrete excessive amounts of urine
B. have an abmormal function of the pancreas
C. both
D. neither   (9:697)

453. Addison's disease

A. usually has a sudden onset
B. is associated with brown pigmentation of the skin
C. both
D. neither   (9:693)

454. Acromegaly is associated with

A. enlargement of the lower jaw
B. enlargement of the bones of the hands
C. both
D. neither   (9:697)

455. Cushing's syndrome

A. is the opposite of Addison's disease
B. is associated with a low tolerance to carbohydrates
C. both
D. neither   (9:694)

456. A patient with uncomplicated rheumatic fever should receive

A. quinidine
B. atropine
C. both
D. neither   (9:852)

457. Gout

A. is a form of arthritis
B. is caused by the deposit of sodium urate crystals in the joints
C. both
D. neither   (9:850)

458. Treatment for a patient with the gout may include

A. phenylbutazone
B. a high-fat diet
C. both
D. neither   (9:851)

459. Nonunion of fractures may be caused by

A. inadequate fixation
B. interposition of muscle between the fragments
C. both
D. neither   (9:860)

460. Delayed union of fractures can be caused by

A. damage to the blood supply
B. inadequate immobilization
C. both
D. neither   (9:860)

461. Trochanteric fractures of the femur

A. tear the retinacula
B. cause a vascular necrosis
C. both
D. neither   (9:873)

462. Traction is used in order to

A. reduce a fracture
B. maintain the alignment of the bones
C. both
D. neither   (9:859)

463. Suspension traction uses

A. weights
B. pulleys
C. both
D. neither   (9:866)

464. Crutchfield tongs are useful for traction in injuries of

A. the cervical spine
B. the lumbar spine
C. both
D. neither   (9:866)

465. Hyperopia

A. is also called farsightedness

B. results when the eyeball is longer than normal
C. both
D. neither   (9:750)

466. A sty

A. is a gland infection of the lid margins
B. can be treated with warm compresses
C. both
D. neither   (9:761)

467. Chalazion

A. results from obstruction of the duct of a tarsal gland
B. heals spontaneously
C. both
D. neither   (9:761)

468. A cataract

A. is an increase in the intraocular pressure
B. occurs more often in the aged
C. both
D. neither   (9:765)

469. "Pink eye"

A. is caused by staphylococci
B. is highly contagious
C. both
D. neither   (9:761)

470. Intraocular pressure can be measured with

A. an ophthalmoscope
B. an oculometer
C. both
D. neither   (9:752)

471. In blepharitis

A. there is an inflammation of the eyelid
B. there is poor vision
C. both
D. neither   (9:761-62)

472. Surgical procedures used for acute glaucoma include

A. iridectomy

B. extraction of the lens
C. both
D. neither   (9:764)

473. The treatment of chronic, closed angle glaucoma includes

A. pilocarpine
B. homatropine
C. both
D. neither   (9:765)

474. Deafness may be a complication of

A. meningococcal infection
B. mumps
C. both
D. neither   (9:560)

475. Deafness has been seen as a complication in patients receiving

A. penicillin
B. streptomycin
C. both
D. neither   (9:660)

476. Otosclerosis causes deafness due to

A. damage of the auditory nerve
B. stapes fixation
C. both
D. neither   (9:560)

477. In otosclerosis, there is

A. a loss of hearing
B. permanent damage to the auditory nerve
C. both
D. neither   (9:558)

478. Meniere's syndrome is

A. caused by a disturbance at the external ear
B. always a complication of chronic otitis
C. both
D. neither   (9:558)

479. Acute follicular tonsillitis is

A. treated by tonsillectomy

B. usually caused by staphylococcus
C. both
D. neither   (9:542)

480. The treatment for acute laryngitis includes

A. voice rest
B. steam inhalations
C. both
D. neither   (9:545)

481. After laryngectomy, a patient may be able to talk with

A. esophageal speach
B. an artificial larynx
C. both
D. neither   (9:553)

482. Lesions in the pyramidal tract may be indicated by a positive

A. Kernig's sign
B. Babinski's sign
C. both
D. neither   (9:781)

483. A positive Romberg's sign

A. indicates locomotor ataxia
B. is associated with paralysis of the lower extremities
C. both
D. neither   (9:781)

484. A positive Babinski's sign

A. indicates irritation in the meninges
B. is usually associated with syphilis
C. both
D. neither   (9:781)

485. Cerebral edema resulting from injury can be reduced by the administration of

A. morphine
B. urea
C. both
D. neither   (9:808)

486. Parkinson's disease

A. is also called paralysis agitans

B. usually affects young persons
C. both
D. neither   (9:791)

487. Patients with Parkinson's disease

A. have a masklike appearance
B. walk with a peculiar running gait
C. both
D. neither   (9:791)

488. In Parkinson's disease

A. there are pathological changes in the basal ganglia
B. the symptoms improve with the use of artane
C. both
D. neither   (9:791)

489. The precipitating cause of migraine headache is

A. hypertension
B. a constriction and then a dilatation of cerebral arteries
C. both
D. neither   (9:794)

490. Common symptoms of multiple sclerosis include

A. diplopia
B. urinary incontinence
C. both
D. neither   (9:790)

491. Diseases associated with rash include

A. rubella (German measles)
B. common cold
C. both
D. neither   (9:716)

492. Acne vulgaris

A. is a viral disease
B. occurs more often in the aged
C. both
D. neither   (9:712)

493. Psoriasis is

A. contagious
B. a benign disease
C. both
D. neither   (9:716)

494. Psoriasis is

A. transmitted by the toad
B. caused by virus
C. both
D. neither   (9:716)

495. Allergic contact dermatitis can be caused by exposure to

A. poison oak
B. poison ivy
C. both
D. neither   (9:714)

496. Treatment for chronic contact dermatitis includes

A. topical corticosteroids
B. wet compresses
C. both
D. neither   (9:714)

497. Warts are

A. benign lesions
B. caused by virus
C. both
D. neither   (9:713)

498. Herpes zoster is

A. also called shingles
B. caused by streptococcus
C. both
D. neither   (9:714)

499. Herpes zoster

A. causes an eruption with a bandlike distribution
B. is more frequent in females
C. both
D. neither   (9:714)

500. In herpes zoster

A. the incubation period is 2 days

B. there is a painful vesicular eruption
C. both
D. neither   (9:714)

501. Impetigo contagiosa is usually

A. due to streptococcus
B. noted on exposed parts of the body
C. both
D. neither   (9:713)

502. Impetigo contagiosa

A. is a viral infection
B. may be endemic in nurseries
C. both
D. neither   (9:713)

503. A patient with impetigo contagiosa

A. should be isolated
B. may be treated with penicillin
C. both
D. neither   (9:713)

504. Epidermophytosis is

A. spread through the use of public showers and swimming pools
B. a fungus infection
C. both
D. neither   (9:711)

505. Tinea barbae is

A. a superficial fungus infection
B. treated with ammoniated mercury preparations
C. both
D. neither   (9:711)

506. In tinea capitis

A. removal of the hair by forceps speeds recovery
B. the hair grows brittle and breaks
C. both
D. neither   (9:711)

507. Leukoplakia

A. occurs on the mucous membranes of the mouth

B. does not need treatment
C. both
D. neither   (9:717)

508. Leukoplakia occurs on

A. the mucous membranes of the mouth
B. the female genitalia
C. both
D. neither   (9:717)

509. Scleroderma

A. usually affects men
B. is a disease in which the skin becomes tight
C. both
D. neither   (9:855)

510. Malignant melanoma has a

A. red color
B. poor prognosis
C. both
D. neither   (9:717)

511. Senile keratoses

A. usually appear in covered parts of the body
B. may undergo malignant degeneration
C. both
D. neither   (9:717)

Directions: Each group of numbered words and statements is followed by the same number of lettered words, phrases or statements. For each numbered word or statement, choose the lettered item that is most closely related to it.

Questions 512 to 516
512. Pneumothorax
513. Bronchiectasis
514. Emphysema
515. Empyema
516. Bronchitis

A. Collection of pus in a preexisting cavity
B. Overdistention of the alveoli
C. Inflammation of the bronchi
D. Dilatation of the bronchial tubes

E. Associated with the presence of air in the pleural space   (9:51,502,514,518)

Questions 517 to 521
517. Pneumonectomy
518. Angiography
519. Plethysmography
520. Lobectomy
521. Thoracoplasty

A. The removal of a lung
B. Removal of one lobe of the lung
C. An extrapleural procedure involving the removal of ribs
D. An aid to diagnosis of peripheral vascular disease
E. An x-ray procedure for the visualization of the heart and blood vessels   (9:345,346,519,520)

Questions 522 to 527
522. Cheyne-Stokes respiration
523. Orthopnea
524. Dyspnea
525. Gavage
526. Incontinence
527. Micturition

A. Shortness of breath
B. Dyspnea occuring after lying down
C. Respiration having periods of apnea and hyperpnea
D. Involuntary expulsion of feces or urine
E. Feeding by tube
F. Act of urinating   (9:41,94,140,315)

Questions 528 to 532
528. Achalasia
529. Dysphagia
530. Fistula
531. Hematemesis
532. Atelectasis

A. Vomiting of blood
B. Difficulty in swallowing food
C. Absence of peristalsis of the esophagus
D. Blockage of air to a portion of the lung
E. A tube like passage (caused by infection) from a normal body cavity to another organ or cavity
(9:51,183,587,593,600)

Questions 533 to 536
533. Diabetes insipidus
534. Dwarfism
535. Acromegaly
536. Diabetes mellitus

A. Associated with congenital deficiency of the growth hormone
B. Associated with hyperfunction of the anterior lobe of the pituitary
C. Caused by a failure of the posterior lobe of the pituitary
D. Associated with insufficient insulin   (9:674,697)

Questions 537 to 541
537. Addison's disease
538. Basedow's disease
539. Exophthalmos
540. Pheochromocytoma
541. Goiter

A. Hyperthyroidism
B. Enlargement of the thyroid
C. Protrusion of the eyeballs
D. Associated with hypofunction of the adrenal cortex
E. A catecholamine-producing tumor
(9:666-67,692,695)

Questions 542 to 548
542. Polyphagia
543. Oliguria
544. Hematuria
545. Polydipsia
546. Pyuria
547. Anuria
548. Polyuria

A. Total suppression of urine
B. Decrease in normal urinary output
C. Pus in the urine
D. Blood in the urine
E. Increased urine volume
F. Increased thirst
G. Increased appetite   (9:409,423,674)

Questions 549 to 552
549. Hyperglycemia
550. Cystitis
551. Glycosuria
552. Litholapaxy

A. Sugar in the urine

B. Increase in blood sugar
C. Procedure by which bladder stones are crushed with a special instrument
D. Inflammation of the lining of the urinary bladder   (9:403,407,674)

Questions 553 to 557
553. Urea clearance test
554. Regitine test
555. Cephalin-cholesterol flocculation test
556. Papanicolaou test
557. Quantitative van den Bergh test

A. Used for the detection of cancer
B. Used for the detection of pheochromocytoma
C. Measures the efficiency of the glomerular filtration of plasma
D. Used to distinguish jaundice due to disease of the liver from obstructive jaundice
E. Measures the total serum bilirubin in the blood   (9:387,441,633,695)

Questions 558 to 562
558. Metrorrhagia
559. Amenorrhea
560. Dysmenorrhea
561. Menorrhagia
562. Leukorrhea

A. Painful menstruation
B. Absence of menstruation
C. Profuse menstrual flow during the regular period
D. Bleeding between periods
E. A white vaginal discharge (9:448,451)

Questions 563 to 568
563. Oophorectomy
564. Colporrhaphy
565. Cystocele
566. Salpingectomy
567. Colpocele
568. Rectocele

A. Repair of the vaginal wall
B. Removal of the fallopian tube
C. Removal of the ovary
D. Prolapse of the vaginal mucosa
E. Herniation of the bladder into the vagina

F. Herniation of the rectal wall into the vagina   (9:457,467)

Questions 569 to 575
569. Presbyopia
570. Astigmatism
571. Ametropia
572. Accomodation
573. Hyperopia
574. Emmetropia
575. Myopia

A. Refers to a normal eye
B. Indicates that a refractive error is present
C. The ability to adjust vision from near to far objects
D. Nearsightedness
E. Farsightedness
F. Caused by asymmetry of the cornea
G. Inability to accommodate to near and far vision   (9:750)

Questions 576 to 580
576. Retrolental fibroplasia
577. Cataract
578. Aphakia
579. Glaucoma
580. Orthoptics

A. Characterized by increased introcular pressure
B. Characterized by clouding of the lens
C. Absence of the crystalline lens
D. A disease of premature infants
E. A technique of exercises used to train a person to use the two eyes together   (9:763,764,765,766)

Questions 581 to 585
581. Hordeolum
582. Keratoplasty
583. Blepharitis
584. Squint
585. Chalazion

A. Inability of the eyes to move simultaneously in the same direction
B. Restoration of a damaged cornea graft
C. Infection of the lid margin
D. A cyst of the eyelid
E. Inflammation of the eyelid (9:761-763)

Questions 586 to 590

586. Paraplegia
587. Akinesia
588. Hemiplegia
589. Quadriplegia
590. Paralgesia

    A. Paralysis of one-half of the body
    B. Paralysis of the lower half of the body
    C. Paralysis of the trunk and all four extremities
    D. Indicates a painful sensation
    E. The loss of a muscle   (9:782)

Questions 591 to 595

591. Macule
592. Papule
593. Vesicle
594. Pustule
595. Bulla

    A. Papule filled with clear fluid
    B. A circumscribed area containing pus
    C. A circumscribed discolored area, not causing skin elevation
    D. A circumscribed elevated skin area
    E. A large elevation of outer skin layers containing serous or purulent fluid   (9:709-710)

Questions 596 to 600

596. Benedict test
597. Sulkowitch test
598. Wasserman test
599. Ketostix
600. Thorn test

    A. Used to test urine for sugar
    B. Used to test urine for acetone
    C. A test for syphilis
    D. Determines the calcium content of the urine
    E. Used to detect inadequate adrenocortical hormone secretion
    (9:395,475,677,784)

Answer Key: Medical-Surgical Nursing

1. C	51. A	101. D	151. C	201. D	251. D	301. A	351. A
2. D	52. D	102. A	152. A	202. C	252. B	302. E	352. A
3. C	53. B	103. A	153. D	203. A	253. B	303. D	353. D
4. C	54. C	104. B	154. B	204. D	254. D	304. A	354. D
5. B	55. B	105. B	155. C	205. D	255. C	305. A	355. D
6. D	56. E	106. C	156. D	206. B	256. B	306. A	356. A
7. C	57. A	107. B	157. B	207. B	257. A	307. B	357. D
8. B	58. C	108. A	158. D	208. A	258. D	308. C	358. C
9. C	59. E	109. B	159. D	209. D	259. A	309. A	359. A
10. A	60. E	110. B	160. A	210. A	260. B	310. D	360. A
11. C	61. D	111. D	161. C	211. C	261. C	311. C	361. D
12. D	62. A	112. D	162. C	212. C	262. D	312. D	362. D
13. D	63. C	113. D	163. D	213. B	263. A	313. D	363. C
14. C	64. D	114. D	164. B	214. D	264. D	314. C	364. C
15. C	65. C	115. A	165. D	215. D	265. D	315. B	365. A
16. C	66. B	116. D	166. D	216. D	266. D	316. D	366. A
17. C	67. D	117. D	167. B	217. D	267. C	317. C	367. D
18. C	68. B	118. D	168. A	218. A	268. D	318. D	368. B
19. B	69. A	119. D	169. C	219. D	269. D	319. B	369. A
20. B	70. C	120. B	170. B	220. D	270. D	320. A	370. B
21. A	71. B	121. C	171. C	221. C	271. A	321. A	371. A
22. A	72. C	122. C	172. D	222. C	272. D	322. D	372. A
23. D	73. A	123. D	173. C	223. D	273. B	323. D	373. C
24. A	74. A	124. D	174. C	224. D	274. D	324. D	374. C
25. D	75. D	125. D	175. B	225. A	275. D	325. C	375. C
26. B	76. D	126. D	176. C	226. A	276. C	326. A	376. A
27. C	77. D	127. A	177. A	227. D	277. B	327. A	377. C
28. C	78. B	128. B	178. A	228. D	278. C	328. D	378. B
29. A	79. C	129. C	179. D	229. A	279. A	329. B	379. C
30. C	80. D	130. D	180. D	230. B	280. B	330. D	380. C
31. D	81. B	131. D	181. D	231. B	281. C	331. D	381. B
32. D	82. A	132. A	182. B	232. D	282. D	332. C	382. B
33. D	83. C	133. B	183. D	233. D	283. C	333. C	383. C
34. D	84. C	134. C	184. D	234. D	284. B	334. B	384. A
35. C	85. A	135. B	185. B	235. B	285. A	335. B	385. B
36. A	86. C	136. B	186. B	236. D	286. A	336. C	386. C
37. A	87. A	137. A	187. D	237. B	287. C	337. D	387. C
38. A	88. C	138. C	188. D	238. D	288. C	338. B	388. C
39. D	89. D	139. C	189. D	239. D	289. A	339. B	389. A
40. C	90. B	140. D	190. D	240. A	290. C	340. D	390. C
41. B	91. D	141. D	191. D	241. B	291. D	341. A	391. D
42. D	92. D	142. D	192. D	242. A	292. C	342. D	392. C
43. D	93. C	143. B	193. B	243. D	293. C	343. D	393. A
44. D	94. E	144. C	194. C	244. D	294. D	344. B	394. C
45. C	95. A	145. A	195. A	245. A	295. B	345. D	395. D
46. D	96. D	146. D	196. D	246. C	296. C	346. A	396. C
47. C	97. C	147. C	197. D	247. D	297. C	347. B	397. C
48. C	98. A	148. A	198. A	248. C	298. C	348. D	398. A
49. C	99. D	149. B	199. A	249. C	299. C	349. D	399. A
50. D	100. D	150. D	200. D	250. D	300. B	350. C	400. C

401. C	426. D	451. C	476. B	501. C	526. D	551. A	576. D
402. C	427. A	452. A	477. A	502. B	527. F	552. C	577. B
403. A	428. A	453. B	478. D	503. C	528. C	553. C	578. C
404. C	429. C	454. C	479. D	504. C	529. B	554. B	579. A
405. B	430. B	455. C	480. C	505. C	530. E	555. D	580. E
406. C	431. C	456. D	481. C	506. C	531. A	556. A	581. C
407. C	432. C	457. C	482. B	507. A	532. D	557. E	582. B
408. B	433. A	458. A	483. A	508. C	533. C	558. D	583. E
409. C	434. C	459. C	484. D	509. B	534. A	559. B	584. A
410. C	435. B	460. C	485. B	510. B	535. B	560. A	585. D
411. B	436. A	461. D	486. A	511. B	536. D	561. C	586. B
412. C	437. C	462. C	487. C	512. E	537. D	562. E	587. E
413. A	438. B	463. C	488. C	513. D	538. A	563. C	588. A
414. C	439. A	464. A	489. B	514. B	539. C	564. A	589. C
415. C	440. B	465. A	490. C	515. A	540. E	565. E	590. D
416. B	441. C	466. C	491. A	516. C	541. B	566. B	591. C
417. C	442. C	467. A	492. D	517. A	542. G	567. D	592. D
418. C	443. D	468. B	493. B	518. E	543. B	568. F	593. A
419. C	444. D	469. B	494. D	519. D	544. D	569. G	594. B
420. D	445. A	470. D	495. C	520. B	545. F	570. F	595. E
421. A	446. A	471. A	496. C	521. C	546. C	571. B	596. A
422. A	447. D	472. A	497. C	522. C	547. A	572. C	597. D
423. D	448. C	473. A	498. A	523. B	548. E	573. E	598. C
424. C	449. C	474. C	499. A	524. A	549. B	574. A	599. B
425. C	450. D	475. B	500. B	525. E	550. D	575. D	600. E

Chapter Six

Psychiatry

Directions: Select from among the lettered choices the one that most appropriately answers the question or completes the statement.

1. A boy hates his father and is torn between the desire to hit him and the fear of the consequences, so he develops a paralyzed arm. This reaction represents an example of

   A. conversion
   B. sublimation
   C. identification
   D. all of the above (12:30)

2. A nurse is angry at her supervisor. In order to let her emotions out, she snaps at her patient. This reaction represents

   A. symbolization
   B. displacement
   C. projection
   D. none of the above (12:32)

3. The mind consists of

   A. the conscious
   B. the subconscious
   C. the unconscious
   D. all of the above (12:34)

4. The founder of the psychoanalytic movement was

   A. Sigmund Freud
   B. Mesmer
   C. Adler
   D. Sullivan (12:35)

5. The founder of the school of individual psychology was

   A. Horney
   B. Phillipe Pinel
   C. Alfred Adler
   D. Dorothea Dix (12:38)

6. Carl Jung identified which of the following functions of the personality?

   A. sensation
   B. intuition
   C. feeling
   D. all of the above (12:40)

7. The founder of the school of analytic psychology was

   A. Freud
   B. Jung
   C. Kraeplin
   D. Meyer (12:40)

8. Projective disorders characteristically occur in

   A. male children
   B. middle-aged persons
   C. old people
   D. teenagers (12:167)

9. A tendency to develop projective techniques of adjustment is found in persons whose childhood produced

   A. hatred
   B. chronic insecurity

115

C. suspiciousness
D. all of the above (12:167)

10. Anxiety neurosis may cause manifestations from the

A. cardiovascular system
B. genitourinary system
C. respiratory system
D. all of the above (12:182)

11. A sociopath has

A. emotional immaturity
B. inability to profit from experience
C. poorly integrated sex life
D. all of the above (12:205)

12. Sociopathic behavior may be due to defective personality development in the area of

A. ego development
B. superego development
C. id development
D. sexual development (12:204)

13. Psychotherapeutic methods include

A. insulin shock
B. electroshock
C. use of tranquilizing drugs
D. all of the above (12:210)

14. The era of shock treatment began in

A. 1860
B. 1912
C. 1933
D. 1952 (12:210)

15. The amount of insulin required to produce therapeutic coma is

A. 60 units
B. 300 units
C. 4,000 units
D. variable (12:211)

16. A danger signal in insulin coma treatment is

A. incontinence of feces
B. convulsions

C. tremor of the extremities
D. perspiration (12:212)

17. Patients remain unconscious after electroshock treatment for

A. several minutes
B. one hour
C. six hours
D. twelve hours (12:216)

18. The most common complication in the use of electroshock therapy is

A. dislocation of the humerus
B. fracture of the femur
C. fracture of the lumbar spine
D. compression fracture of the spine in the middorsal region (12:217)

19. Electroshock therapy is not permitted in patients with

A. cardiac decompensation
B. peptic ulcer
C. diabetes
D. all of the above (12:217)

20. A surgical approach to the treatment of mental illness was begun by

A. Cerletti
B. Egas Moniz
C. Bini
D. Freeman (12:218)

21. Narcoanalysis consists of a very slow intravenous injection of

A. promazine
B. sodium amytal
C. fluphenazine
D. reserpine (12:220)

22. The meprobamates are used in

A. alcoholism
B. petit mal epilepsy
C. anxiety
D. all of the above (12:223)

23. A useful drug in the treatment of schizophrenic patients is

A. diazepam
B. oxazepam
C. hydroxyzine
D. the phenothiazines   (12:223)

24. Patients prepared for electroshock therapy should not be given

    A. antibiotics
    B. vitamin B
    C. major tranquilizers such as chlor-promazine
    D. all of the above   (12:223)

25. All of the following are antidepressant drugs *except*

    A. Tofranil
    B. Elavil
    C. Parnate
    D. Talwin   (12:224)

26. General paresis is a condition caused by

    A. malaria
    B. syphilis
    C. typhoid fever
    D. gonorrhea   (12:247)

27. An aura is seen

    A. in manic reaction
    B. in paranoid reaction
    C. in involutional reaction
    D. by the epileptic preceding seizure   (12:248)

28. A disturbance in consciousness is seen in all of the following *except*

    A. Huntington's chorea
    B. petit mal
    C. grand mal
    D. psychomotor epileptic equivalents   (12:248,250)

29. Convulsive phenomena can be seen in

    A. cerebral arteriosclerosis
    B. meningitis
    C. uremia
    D. all of the above   (12:248)

30. Huntington's chorea causes impairment of

    A. memory
    B. attention
    C. judgement
    D. all of the above   (12:250)

31. Drugs used in the treatment of petit mal attacks include

    A. trimethadione
    B. paramethadione
    C. phensuximine
    D. all of the above   (12:250)

32. All of the following are used in the treatment of grand mal *except*

    A. phenobarbital
    B. diphenylhydantoin
    C. penicillin
    D. phenantoin   (12:250)

33. The treatment of behavior disorders with convulsions is based on

    A. regulation of diet
    B. medication to control seizures
    C. environmental adjustment
    D. all of the above   (12:250)

34. All of the following can be used for the control of the physical symptoms of Parkinson's disease *except*

    A. profenamine
    B. orphenadrine
    C. cycrimine
    D. benzedrine   (12:251)

35. Mental retardation can be caused by

    A. meningitis
    B. encephalitis
    C. brain abscess
    D. all of the above   (12:311)

36. The hebephrenic type of schizophrenia is characterized by

    A. mannerisms
    B. giggling
    C. regressive behavior
    D. all of the above   (12:329)

37. Involutional melancholia is characterized by all of the following *except*

    A. agitation
    B. worry
    C. convulsions
    D. insomnia   (12:330)

38. The manic type of manic depressive illness is associated with

    A. flight of ideas
    B. accelerated speech
    C. accelerated motor activity
    D. all of the above   (12:330)

39. Asthenic personality is characterized by

    A. insensitivity to emotional stress
    B. increased enthusiasm
    C. marked capacity for enjoyment
    D. all of the above
    E. none of the above   (12:332)

40. Which of the following illnesses does not have a psychophysiologic origin?
    A. bronchial asthma
    B. ulcerative colitis
    C. peptic ulcer
    D. erysipelas   (12:334)

41. Antidepressant drugs

    A. lift the mood
    B. calm disturbed behavior
    C. restore vitality
    D. all of the above   (12:337)

42. When a patient is unable to control a repetitive behavior that he considers illogical, he exhibits

    A. phobia
    B. compulsion
    C. imagination
    D. projection   (12:338)

43. The direction of interests and emotions toward one's self is called

    A. insight

    B. identification
    C. introversion
    D. none of the above   (12:339)

44. The id, as formulated by Freud,

    A. is a term used to denote the unconscious part of the personality
    B. contains primitive urges
    C. is ruled by the pleasure principle
    D. all of the above   (12:339)

45. A misinterpreted sensory perception is called

    A. illusion
    B. delusion
    C. insight
    D. all of the above   (12:339)

46. A morbid fear of disease germs is called

    A. transference
    B. suppression
    C. phobia
    D. repression   (12:340)

47. The hebephrenic type of schizophrenia is characterized by

    A. bizarre delusions
    B. hallucinations
    C. silliness
    D. all of the above   (12:342)

48. In the simple type of schizophrenia, there is

    A. blunting of emotion
    B. childlike behavior
    C. apathy
    D. all of the above   (12:342)

49. The following are types of schizophrenia *except* the

    A. catatonic type
    B. paranoid type
    C. stuttering type
    D. hebephrenic type   (12:342)

50. Waxy flexibility is found in

    A. stuttering

B. porencephaly
C. catatonic schizophrenia
D. all of the above   (12:342)

51. Ventilation means free verbal expression of
    A. feelings
    B. tension
    C. problems
    D. all of the above   (12:342)

Answer the questions in this group by following the directions below. Select

    A. if only A is correct
    B. if only B is correct
    C. if both A and B are correct
    D. if both A and B are incorrect

52. Anxiety can be aroused by
    A. external danger
    B. internal danger
    C. both
    D. neither   (12:25)

53. Attempts to give "morale treatment" to the mentally ill were made early in France by

    A. Dr. Philippe Pinel
    B. Erik Erikson
    C. both
    D. neither   (12:5)

54. In ancient times mentally ill persons were considered to be

    A. superstitious
    B. under the influence of evil spirits
    C. both
    D. neither   (12:5)

55. The mental mechanism of conversion is strongly influenced by

    A. cultural factors
    B. nutritional factors
    C. both
    D. neither   (12:30)

56. Mental mechanisms operating on an unconscious level include

    A. repression

B. conversion
C. both
D. neither   (12:30)

57. The concept of the unconscious was popularized by

    A. Freud
    B. Adler
    C. both
    D. neither   (12:34)

58. Psychoanalytic groups agree to which of the following?

    A. behavior is not determined by chance
    B. all behavior is goal-directed
    C. both
    D. neither   (12:43)

59. The name of Harry Stack Sullivan is connected with the

    A. interpersonal theory of psychiatry
    B. technique of free association
    C. both
    D. neither   (12:42)

60. In patients with protective patterns, the major mechanism of adjustment is

    A. projection
    B. acceptance of reality
    C. both
    D. neither   (12:167)

61. Anxiety neurosis may be accompanied by

    A. discouragement
    B. difficulty in remembering
    C. both
    D. neither   (12:182)

62. Treatment for anxiety neurosis includes

    A. electroshock therapy
    B. psychotherapy
    C. both
    D. neither   (12:185)

63. The nurse should be able to understand

    A. what she can do for a neurotic patient

B. what she cannot do for a neurotic patient
C. both
D. neither (12:188)

64. Patients with anxiety neurosis should

A. develop recreational skills
B. participate in activities with others
C. both
D. neither (12:188)

65. The nurse can help a patient with anxiety neurosis by providing

A. reassurance
B. encouragement
C. both
D. neither (12:188)

66. Sociopathic personality is associated with

A. psychotic symptoms
B. social agression
C. both
D. neither (12:205)

67. Patients with sociopathic personality have

A. superficial charm
B. antisocial attitude
C. both
D. neither (12:204)

68. Sociopaths very often suffer from

A. remorse
B. shame
C. both
D. neither (12:205)

69. Sociopaths may not be able to profit by psychotherapy because of inability to

A. integrate new experiences
B. alter their personality development through corrective experience
C. both
D. neither (12:207)

70. Insulin coma produced for therapeutic reasons can be terminated by the administration of

A. sugar
B. protamine
C. both
D. neither (12:211)

71. Complications occurring in the use of insulin shock therapy include

A. cardiac collapse
B. irreversible coma
C. both
D. neither (12:212)

72. Nursing care during insulin shock treatment includes

A. avoiding insulin injection into fatty surface tissue
B. observation of the patient for signs of allergic response to insulin
C. both
D. neither (12:213)

73. Insulin shock treatment is effective in treating

A. general paresis
B. withdrawal patterns of behavior
C. both
D. neither (12:212)

74. Insulin shock treatment

A. is an adjunct to psychiatric therapy
B. helps to reduce the length of hospitalization
C. both
D. neither (12:212)

75. During electroshock treatment, the patient shows

A. tonic spasms
B. clonic spasms
C. both
D. neither (12:216)

76. Electroshock therapy is contraindicated in

A. coronary thrombosis
B. unhealed bone fractures
C. both
D. neither (12:217)

77. Electroshock treatment is effective in

    A. paranoid type of schizophrenia
    B. catatonic type of schizophrenia
    C. both
    D. neither   (12:217)

78. Psychosurgery was introduced in the United States by

    A. Freeman and Watts
    B. Manfred Sakel
    C. both
    D. neither   (12:218)

79. There is evidence of a relationship between behavior and the level of

    A. potent amines in the brain
    B. serum cholesterol
    C. both
    D. neither   (12:221)

80. Tranquilizers calm the patient by

    A. reducing anxiety
    B. disturbing psychotic behavior
    C. both
    D. neither   (12:221)

81. A patient with anxiety receiving a minor tranquilizer may manifest

    A. autonomic side effects
    B. extrapyramidal side affects
    C. both
    D. neither   (12:223)

82. Major tranquilizers include

    A. perphenazine
    B. diazepam
    C. both
    D. neither   (12:222)

83. Minor tranquilizers include

    A. haloperidol
    B. promizine
    C. both
    D. neither   (12:222)

84. Antidepressant drugs affect

    A. mood
    B. behavior
    C. both
    D. neither   (12:224)

85. Acute organic behavior disorders can be caused by

    A. an overdose of barbiturates
    B. prolonged ingestion of bromides
    C. both
    D. neither   (12:240)

86. Behavior disorders are seen in

    A. cerebral arteriosclerosis
    B. general paresis
    C. both
    D. neither   (12:246-47)

87. General paresis is associated with infection of

    A. the meninges
    B. the cerebellum
    C. both
    D. neither   (12:247)

88. The pupils of patients with general paresis may be

    A. contracted
    B. unequal
    C. both
    D. neither   (12:247)

89. The Argyll-Robertson pupil seen in general paresis reacts to

    A. light
    B. accommodation
    C. both
    D. neither   (12:247)

90. Convulsive phenomena may be seen in

    A. idiopathic epilepsy
    B. lead poisoning
    C. both
    D. neither   (12:248)

91. A very brief loss of consciousness characterizes

A. petit mal attacks
B. Parkinson's disease
C. both
D. neither   (12:249)

92. In grand mal seizures

A. loss of consciousness takes place first
B. a tonic spasm follows the loss of consciousness
C. both
D. neither   (12:249)

93. Behavior changes can be seen in

A. the period following epidemic encephalitis
B. Huntington's chorea
C. both
D. neither   (12:250)

94. Huntington's chorea

A. is characterized by irregular movements
B. renders the patient unable to carry out normal activities
C. both
D. neither   (12:250)

95. Huntington's chorea

A. results from degeneration of specific areas in the brain
B. makes custodial detention necessary for the patient
C. both
D. neither   (12:250)

96. Patients with Huntington's chorea are

A. irritable
B. emotionally labile
C. both
D. neither   (12:250)

97. Heredity is the chief etiologic factor in

A. Huntington's chorea
B. anxiety
C. both
D. neither   (12:250)

98. Persons who drink excessively do so because

A. alcohol provides temporary relief from emotional tension
B. alcohol speeds up the brain action
C. both
D. neither   (12:260)

99. Disulfiram (Antabuse), a drug used in the treatment of alcoholism, is effective because it

A. destroys the taste for alcohol
B. increases the tolerance for alcohol
C. both
D. neither   (12:263)

100. An alcoholic patient can be helped by

A. electroshock therapy
B. psychotherapy guiding the patient to understand his problems
C. both
D. neither   (12:264)

101. When dealing with an alcoholic patient, the nurse should

A. have an attitude of understanding
B. explain to him that he must be ashamed about his drinking
C. both
D. neither   (12:265)

102. When dealing with an alcoholic patient, the nurse should try to

A. stimulate interest in his family
B. help him to feel accepted
C. both
D. neither   (2:265)

103. Physical dependence can be caused by

A. marihuana
B. cocaine
C. both
D. neither   (12:274,275)

104. Drugs that can cause physical dependence include

A. opium
B. amphetamines
C. both
D. neither   (12:271,275)

105. Psychologic dependence can be caused by

A. opium
B. cocaine
C. both
D. neither   (12:271)

106. The drug abuser is often described as

A. insecure
B. immature
C. both
D. neither   (12:279)

107. Breath-holding in infants may be an expression of

A. resentment
B. frustration
C. both
D. neither   (12:295)

108. The catatonic type of schizophrenia is associated with

A. mutism
B. negativism
C. both
D. neither   (12:329)

109. Frequent symptoms of the simple type of schizophrenia include

A. delusions
B. hallucinations
C. both
D. neither   (12:329)

110. Patients suffering from neuroses have

A. gross personality disorganization
B. gross distortion of reality
C. both
D. neither   (12:331)

111. Affective disorders include

A. involutional melancholia

B. manic-depressive illness
C. both
D. neither   (12:330)

112. The depressed phase of manic-depressive illness is characterized by

A. mental retardation
B. motor retardation
C. both
D. neither   (12:330)

113. Disturbed behavior characterizes

A. schizophrenia
B. paranoid states
C. both
D. neither   (12:331)

114. In the paranoid state, there is a disturbance in

A. mood
B. thinking
C. both
D. neither   (12:331)

115. Depersonalization neurosis is characterized by

A. a feeling of unreality
B. fear of disease of various organs
C. both
D. neither   (12:332)

116. Neurasthenic neurosis is associated with

A. chronic weakness
B. easy fatigability
C. both
D. neither   (12:332)

117. Asthenic personality is characterized by

A. low energy level
B. oversensitivity to physical stress
C. both
D. neither   (12:332)

118. Psychophysiologic respiratory disorders include

A. hyperventilation syndrome

B. pneumonia alba
C. both
D. neither   (12:334)

119. Psychophysiologic musculoskeletal disorders include

A. tension headache
B. rheumatic fever
C. both
D. neither   (12:334)

120. Anxiety may be caused by

A. real danger
B. imagined danger
C. both
D. neither   (12:337)

121. Delirium is characterized by

A. confusion
B. disordered speech
C. both
D. neither   (12:338)

122. In hypochondriasis, there is a morbid preoccupation with

A. persons of the opposite sex
B. the state of health
C. both
D. neither   (12:339)

123. Hysteria is

A. a psychoneurosis
B. characterized by absence of physical symptoms
C. both
D. neither   (12:339)

124. In neurasthenia, there is

A. motor fatigability
B. mental fatigability
C. both
D. neither   (12:340)

125. Patients with the catatonic type of schizophrenia show

A. phases of stupor

B. phases of excitement
C. both
D. neither   (12:342)

126. Schizophrenia is characterized by lack of correlation between

A. thinking and feeling
B. experience and reality
C. both
D. neither   (12:342)

Each statement is followed by four suggested answers. Answer according to the following key:

A. **if 1, 2, and 3 are correct**
B. **if 1 and 3 are correct**
C. **if 2 and 4 are correct**
D. **if only 4 is correct**
E. **if all are correct**

127. Anxiety neurosis symptoms may include
1. headache
2. marked sensitivity to sensory stimulation
3. difficulty in concentrating
4. irritability   (12:182)

128. Sociopathic behavior is characterized by
1. good judgment
2. amorality
3. increased capacity for remorse
4. explosiveness under pressure (12:205)

129. Patients with sociopathic personalities are characterized by
1. high intelligence
2. sense of responsibility
3. insincerity
4. altruism   (12:204)

130. In working with a sociopath, the nurse should be
1. friendly
2. cautious
3. consistent
4. indulgent   (12:207)

131. Care during insulin shock treatment includes

　　1. keeping the patient covered with blankets
　　2. use of suction if the throat must be cleared
　　3. keeping the patients head turned to the side
　　4. taking a blood specimens for a blood count　　　　(12:213)

132. Reactions to insulin shock therapy include

　　1. weakness
　　2. excessive perspiration
　　3. tremor
　　4. insomnia　　　　(12:212)

133. Electroshock treatment calls for electrodes on the patient's

　　1. arms
　　2. chest
　　3. thighs
　　4. temples　　　　(12:216)

134. Electroshock therapy is effective in

　　1. agitated depression
　　2. hysterical neurosis
　　3. retarded depression
　　4. schizophrenia　　　　(12:216)

135. Surgical procedures used in selective treatment of mental illness include

　　1. prefrontal lobotomy
　　2. topectomy
　　3. thalamotomy
　　4. transorbital lobotomy　　　　(12:218)

136. Major tranquilizers include

　　1. rescinnamine
　　2. prochlorperazine
　　3. trifluoperazine
　　4. adiphenine　　　　(12:223)

137. Minor tranquilizers include

　　1. deserpidine
　　2. thioridazine

3. perphenazine
4. mephenesin　　　　(12:222)

138. A tranquilizing action is produced by

　　1. meprobamate
　　2. aluminum phosphate
　　3. mepazine
　　4. picrotoxin　　　　(12:222)

139. Patients with general paresis may show

　　1. tremor of the face
　　2. disturbance of speech
　　3. changes in handwriting
　　4. absent deep tendon reflexes　(12:247)

140. Symptoms of delirium tremens include

　　1. visual hallucinations
　　2. marked tremor
　　3. ataxia
　　4. motor restlessness　　　　(12:262)

141. Inadequate personality is characterized by ineffectual response to

　　1. physical demands
　　2. emotional demands
　　3. intellectual demands
　　4. social demands　　　　(12:333)

142. Patients with antisocial personalities are

　　1. callous
　　2. impulsive
　　3. incapable of loyalty
　　4. unable to learn from punishment　　　　(12:332)

143. Hysterical personality is characterized by

　　1. self-dramatization
　　2. overreactivity
　　3. excitability
　　4. emotional stability　　　　(12:332)

144. Psychophysiologic skin disorders include

　　1. atopic dermatitis
　　2. impetigo
　　3. neurodermatosis
　　4. herpes　　　　(12:334)

145. Withdrawing reaction is characterized by

    1. seclusiveness
    2. detachment
    3. shyness
    4. inability to form close relationships (12:335)

146. Features of grand mal include

    1. tonic spasms
    2. a series of jerky movements
    3. loss of consciousness
    4. hallucinations (12:339)

147. Delirium tremens is associated with prolonged use of

    1. barbiturates
    2. tranquilizers
    3. antidepressants
    4. alcohol (12:338)

148. Dementia praecox is a term used to indicate

    1. Alzhiemer's disease
    2. epilepsy
    3. Korsakoff's psychosis
    4. schizophrenia (12:388)

149. Features of Korsakoff's psychosis include

    1. acute illness
    2. the use of alcohol
    3. increased intellectual capacities
    4. polyneuritis (12:340)

Directions: Each group of numbered words and statements is followed by the same number of lettered words, phrases or statements. For each numbered word or statement, choose the lettered item that is most closely related to it.

Questions 150 to 152

150. The child learns to enjoy eliminative functions

151. Feeding at the breast is source of greatest pleasure

152. Source of pleasure is deflected to the genital region

    A. Oral stage
    B. Anal stage
    C. Phallic stage (12:34,36)

Questions 153 to 155
153. Insulin therapy
154. Group therapy
155. Electroshock therapy

    A. Coma produced by gradually increased doses of insulin
    B. Electric current applied to the brain
    C. Assists patients to adjust to group living situations (12:121,213,216)

Questions 156 to 160
156. Characterized by self-dramatization
157. Recurring periods of depression and elation
158. Characterized by seclusiveness and avoidance of competitive relationships
159. Characterized by excessive concern with conformity
160. Characterized by rigidity, hypersensitivity, jealousy

    A. Paranoid personality
    B. Cyclothymic personality
    C. Obsessive compulsive personality
    D. Schizoid personality
    E. Hysterical personality (12:332)

Questions 161 to 165
161. Addiction
162. Amnesia
163. Aberration
164. Agression
165. Anxiety

    A. Deviation from what is normal or natural
    B. Psychological and physical dependence upon a drug
    C. A feeling or action that is hostile or self-assertive
    D. A loss of memory
    E. A state of apprehensive tension (12:337)

Questions 166 to 170
166. Hallucination
167. Epilepsy
168. Mutism
169. Narcissism
170. Negativism

    A. A disturbance in consciousness that may be accompanied by convulsions
    B. An imaginary sense perception
    C. The inability to speak
    D. A term denoting self love
    E. A generalized resistance to any suggestion from outside the self

    (12:339,340)

Questions 171 to 175
171. Delusion
172. Depression
173. Deterioration
174. Euphoria
175. Dementia

    A. A deterioration of intellectual capacities
    B. A feeling of sadness or dejection
    C. A fixed false belief that cannot be corrected by reason or evidence
    D. An impairment in quality or character
    E. An exaggerated sense of well being

    (12:338,339)

Questions 176 to 180
176. Apathy
177. Congruence
178. Empathy
179. Confabulation
180. Autism

    A. Consistency in thinking, feeling, and actions
    B. The filling in of memory gaps with made-up episodes
    C. The capacity of feeling in communion with others
    D. A state of indifference
    E. An introspective absorption in fantasy with a complete exclusion of reality

    (12:337,338)

Questions 181 to 184
181. Blocking
182. Displacement
183. Blunting
184. Compulsion

    A. Sudden stoppage in the stream of thought
    B. Dullness of emotional response
    C. An uncontrollable urge to think or act against one's better judgment
    D. A mechanism whereby the emotions associated with one idea or object are unconsciously attached to another

    (12:337,338)

Questions 185 to 188
185. Extroversion
186. Conversion
187. Identification
188. Obsession

    A. The uncontrollable urge to think some thought against one's will
    B. A mechanism by which one feels or thinks as another person
    C. The direction of interest and emotions toward the environment
    D. The process by which an emotional conflict is expressed as a physical symptom   (12:338,339)

Questions 189 to 193
189. Pica
190. Insight
191. Phobia
192. Libido
193. Repression

    A. A compulsive fear
    B. The habitual ingestion of substances that have no nutritional value
    C. The vital force that motivates living
    D. A reasonably accurate selfjudgement
    E. A mental mechanism that keeps from awareness unpleasant experiences

    (12:339-41)

Questions 194 to 197
194. Regression
195. Sublimation
196. Reaction
197. Suppression

    A. The state of refusing to accept
    B. Reversion to patterns of behavior characteristic of an earlier phase of development

C. A mental mechanism whereby the energy associated with primitive drives is utilized in constructive social activities

D. A mental mechanism whereby unpleasant feelings and experiences are kept from awareness   (12:341,342)

Questions 198 to 200

198. Unconscious
199. Symbolization
200. Superego

    A. The critical aspect of the personality
    B. The investment of one idea in another
    C. The part of mental activity that is not accessible to conscious awareness

                    (12:338,342)

Answer Key: Psychiatry

1. A	26. B	51. D	76. C	101. A	126. C	151. A	176. D
2. B	27. D	52. C	77. D	102. B	127. E	152. C	177. A
3. D	28. A	53. A	78. A	103. D	128. C	153. A	178. C
4. A	29. D	54. B	79. A	104. C	129. B	154. C	179. B
5. C	30. D	55. A	80. C	105. C	130. A	155. B	180. E
6. D	31. D	56. C	81. D	106. C	131. A	156. E	181. A
7. B	32. C	57. A	82. A	107. C	132. A	157. B	182. D
8. B	33. D	58. C	83. D	108. C	133. D	158. D	183. B
9. D	34. D	59. A	84. C	109. D	134. B	159. C	184. C
10. D	35. D	60. A	85. C	110. D	135. E	160. A	185. C
11. D	36. D	61. C	86. C	111. C	136. A	161. B	186. D
12. B	37. C	62. B	87. A	112. C	137. D	162. D	187. B
13. D	38. D	63. C	88. C	113. C	138. B	163. A	188. A
14. C	39. E	64. C	89. B	114. C	139. E	164. C	189. B
15. D	40. D	65. C	90. C	115. A	140. E	165. E	190. D
16. B	41. D	66. B	91. A	116. C	141. E	166. B	191. A
17. A	42. B	67. C	92. D	117. C	142. E	167. A	192. C
18. D	43. C	68. D	93. C	118. A	143. A	168. C	193. E
19. A	44. D	69. C	94. C	119. A	144. B	169. D	194. B
20. B	45. A	70. A	95. C	120. C	145. E	170. E	195. C
21. B	46. C	71. C	96. C	121. C	146. A	171. C	196. A
22. D	47. D	72. C	97. A	122. B	147. D	172. B	197. D
23. D	48. D	73. B	98. A	123. A	148. D	173. D	198. C
24. C	49. C	74. C	99. A	124. C	149. C	174. E	199. B
25. D	50. C	75. C	100. B	125. C	150. B	175. A	200. A

Chapter Seven

Nutrition and Diet Therapy

Directions: Select from among the lettered choices the one that most appropriately answers the question or completes the statement.

1. The sweetest sugar is

   A. glucose
   B. lactose
   C. fructose
   D. galactose   (8:42)

2. Ordinary table sugar is

   A. sucrose
   B. glucose
   C. maltose
   D. none of the above   (8:42)

3. Polysaccharides of interest in nutrition include

   A. starch
   B. dextrin
   C. cellulose
   D. all of the above   (8:42)

4. Which is highest in carbohydrate content?

   A. corn
   B. macaroni
   C. carrots
   D. spinach   (8:51)

5. Carbohydrates can be found in

   A. vegetables
   B. fruits
   C. milk
   D. all of the above   (8:49)

6. Animal fat components include

   A. palmitic acid
   B. stearic acid
   C. oleic acid
   D. all of the above   (8:55)

7. Lipids important in nutrition include

   A. lecithin
   B. cephalin
   C. spingomyelins
   D. all of tha above   (8:53)

8. The content of saturated fatty acids is greatest in

   A. butter
   B. corn oil
   C. beef suet
   D. lard   (8:55)

9. Essential fatty acids include

   A. linoleic acid
   B. linolenic acid
   C. arachidonic acid
   D. all of the above   (8:56)

10. How many calories does a gram of fat yield?

   A. 5
   B. 6
   C. 8
   D. 9   (8:56)

11. A negative nitrogen balance occurs when

    A. more nitrogen is being ingested than is excreted in the urine
    B. new tissue is being built in periods of rapid growth
    C. dietary protein intake is adequate for tissue synthesis
    D. the body's energy needs must be met from the body's store of fat and the reserves of protein   (8:69)

12. Excessive putrefaction in the large intestine is usually associated with too much

    A. carbohydrate foods
    B. lactic foods
    C. enzyme fluids
    D. protein foods   (8:93)

13. Assume that a pregnant patient cannot drink milk. The lack of protein can best be compensated for by using greater amounts of

    A. noodles and butter
    B. peanut butter and plums
    C. hamburger and legumes
    D. whole wheat bread and carrots   (8:81)

14. Function of minerals in the body deals with

    A. maintenance of osmotic pressure
    B. maintenance of acid-base balance
    C. maintenance of nerve irritability
    D. all of the above   (8:100)

15. According to the National Research Council, which of the following statements is correct?

    A. the daily protein requirement for a man weighing 65 kgs is 80 g
    B. the daily vitamin A requirement for a pregnant woman is 5000 I.U.
    C. the daily calcium requirement for a woman is 800 mg
    D. the daily iron requirement for a man is 20 mg   (8:103)

16. The effects of calcium and phosphorus insufficiency are first seen in the

    A. red blood corpuscles
    B. thyroid gland

    C. skeletal structure
    D. pancreas   (8:104)

17. When iron is needed in the diet, the best food to supplement with would be

    A. shredded wheat
    B. beef liver
    C. spinach
    D. rhubard   (8:107)

18. When iron is needed in the diet, the poorest food to supplement with would be

    A. peanuts
    B. whole eggs
    C. shredded wheat
    D. white bread   (8:107)

19. The group containing foods highest in iron is

    A. cheese, liver, lean meats
    B. cheese, green leafy vegetables, milk
    C. liver, milk, citrus fruit
    D. liver, green leafy vegetables, lean meats   (8:107)

20. Fish liver oil is an important source of

    A. vitamim B_1
    B. vitamin B_6
    C. vitamin D
    D. vitamin B_{12} (8:125)

21. Insufficient iron in the diet may cause

    A. hypertension
    B. edema of the extremities
    C. pernicious anemia
    D. hypochromic anemia
    E. diabetes   (8:108)

22. Experimental evidence has shown that some dietary factor is a specific in the prevention or correction of all cases of

    A. underweight
    B. arthritis
    C. xerophthalmia
    D. colds   (8:125)

23. A dietary deficiency of fluorine may result in clinical evidence of

    A. dental caries
    B. dermatitis
    C. edema
    D. osteoporosis   (8:113)

24. Vitamin D, which is often added to milk, is an important aid in the prevention of

    A. beriberi
    B. pellagra
    C. rickets
    D. scurvy   (8:126)

25. A condition which is *not* generally the result of a deficiency of absence of vitamin E in the diet is

    A. degeneration of germinal epithelium in the male
    B. death and resorption of developing young
    C. soreness and inflammation of the tongue and mouth
    D. failure of placental function in the female   (8:128)

26. A condition which is not generally the result of a deficiency or absence of vitamin E in the diet is

    A. nervous and mental disorders
    B. sterility
    C. disturbance in gestation
    D. resorption of developing young (8:128)

27. Beriberi is a deficiency disease caused by the lack of

    A. thiamine
    B. vitamin C
    C. vitamin A
    D. vitamin B_1 (8:131)

28. A pyridoxin deficient diet may cause

    A. epileptiform seizures
    B. infertility
    C. osteomalacia
    D. bone fractures   (8:136)

29. Deficiency of biotin causes

    A. dermatitis
    B. loss of hair
    C. muscular incoordination
    D. all of the above   (8:138)

30. A vitamin especially helpful in curing scurvy is

    A. vitamin C
    B. vitamin D
    C. vitamin B
    D. vitamin A   (8:143)

31. Fish liver oil is an important source of

    A. vitamin K
    B. vitamin C
    C. vitamin F
    D. vitamin A   (8:125)

32. Of the following lists of foods, the one which will contribute most to the ascorbic acid content of a diet is

    A. potatoes, green peppers, raw cabbage
    B. enriched bread, pork, turnips
    C. whole wheat bread, potatoes, prunes
    D. apples, dates, plums   (8:147)

33. Minerals maintaining osmotic equilibrium in the body include

    A. sodium
    B. potassium
    C. chloride
    D. all of the above   (8:153)

34. The number of grams of protein that a normal, moderately active woman weighing 133 pounds would require daily is approximately

    A. 40
    B. 60
    C. 90
    D. 70   (8:158)

35. The recommended protein intake for the average adult is 1 gram of protein per kilogram of ideal body weight. On this basis, the protein requirement for an adult who should weigh 140 pounds is

A. 54.6 g
B. 63.5 g
C. 85.9 g
D. 140 g   (8:158)

36. The recommended daily dietary allowance of protein for an aged man is most nearly

    A. 0.5g per kg body weight
    B. 1 g per kg body weight
    C. 1.5 g per kg body weight
    D. 2 g per kg body weight   (8:159)

37. The greatest amount of protein per unit of body weight is needed during

    A. childhood
    B. infancy
    C. adolescence
    D. pregnancy   (8:158)

38. Of the following statements, the one concerning the nutritive requirement for a pregnant woman in the third trimester which is not correct is that the

    A. vitamin A requirement is increased
    B. protein requirement is increased from 55 to 80 g
    C. nutritional requirements can be met on a 1000 caloric diet
    D. calcium requirement is increased (8:241)

39. The daily diet of a pregnant woman of average size should contain at least

    A. 25 g of protein
    B. 50 g of protein
    C. 65 g of protein
    D. 150 g of protein   (8:241)

40. The diet most likely to be ordered for the pernicious vomiting of pregnancy is

    A. high carbohydrate, low fat
    B. high carbohydrate, high fat, high protein
    C. low carbohydrate, low fat, high protein
    D. high protein, low sodium   (8:249)

41. Of the following, the statement concerning the nutritive requirements for lactation which is incorrect is that

    A. 1 to 1.5 quarts of milk are needed daily
    B. the riboflavin requirement is increased
    C. the protein requirement is the same as in pregnancy
    D. the ascorbic acid requirement is increased   (8:241)

42. The type of milk best suited for an infant's diet is

    A. mother's milk
    B. irradiated goat's milk
    C. Grade A pasteurized milk
    D. raw milk heated beyond the boiling point   (8:257)

43. From the point of view of infant feeding, the most digestible of the following types of milk is

    A. raw milk
    B. evaporated milk
    C. pasteurized milk
    D. boiled milk   (8:258)

44. In order to meet the vitamin C requirement, the daily menu for a two-year-old should include at least

    A. 1 cup of orange juice
    B. 1/2 cup of orange juice
    C. 2 glasses of tomato juice
    D. 1 glass of mixed vegetable juice (8:279)

45. The amount of milk per pound of body weight which a baby's formula should include daily in order to furnish the amount of protein necessary for normal growth is

    A. one-half ounce
    B. one ounce
    C. two ounces
    D. four ounces   (8:259)

46. When feeding an aged person, it is usually least desirable to

    A. allow frequent small feedings rather than 3 meals a day
    B. stress refined, easily digested carbohydrate foods
    C. serve hot food at each meal
    D. serve the largest meal of the day at lunch   (8:292)

47. The nutritional needs of older people differ from those of young adults in that older people require more

    A. protein
    B. minerals
    C. calcium
    D. calories (8:294)

48. The normal daily fluid intake for an adult is

    A. 1500 to 2000 cc
    B. 6000 to 8000 cc
    C. 4 to 6 glasses
    D. 1 quart (8:312)

49. The thiamine needs of an individual are dependant upon his

    A. total caloric intake
    B. body weight
    C. body height
    D. age (8:131)

50. The "house diet" is generally best used to indicate the diet for patients

    A. having only a slight fever
    B. having incipient tuberculosis
    C. confined by incapacities other than illness
    D. convalescing from a serious illness (8:315)

51. Of the following, the one *not* ordinarily regarded as a standard hospital diet is a

    A. restricted water diet
    B. restricted-liquid diet
    C. full diet
    D. light diet (8:316)

52. Of the following, the food *not* generally included in a light diet is

    A. mayonnaise
    B. nuts
    C. coarse vegetables
    D. brains (8:317)

53. Of the following, the food *not* generally included in a light diet is

    A. prepared cereal

    B. ground meat
    C. citrus fruit
    D. scraped beef (8:317)

54. Of the following, the food *not* generally included in light diet is

    A. steak
    B. olives
    C. broiled lamb chops
    D. potatoes (8:317)

55. A soft diet is

    A. high in fat
    B. low in residue and readily digested
    C. not readily digested
    D. high in laxative properties (8:318)

56. Of the following groups, the one which may be served on a soft diet is

    A. cream soup, mashed potato, spinach purée, toast, butter, custard
    B. broiled chicken, mashed potato, buttered peas, toast, milk
    C. vegetable soup, lamb chop, mashed potato, lettuce salad, toast
    D. clear broth, baked potato, tenderloin steak, carrots, apple pie (8:318)

57. Of the following, the food which may be generally included in a soft diet is

    A. grated cheese
    B. sweetbreads
    C. soft-cooked eggs
    D. broiled lamb (8:318)

58. Of the following, the food which may generally be included in a soft diet is

    A. milk pudding
    B. broiled bacon
    C. nuts
    D. fish (8:318)

59. Of the following, the food *not* generally included in a soft diet is

    A. fruit juice
    B. mashed potatoes
    C. bran cereal
    D. cottage cheese (8:318)

60. Of the following, the food *not* generally included in a soft diet is

    A. plain, cooked spaghetti
    B. baked potatoes
    C. cooked fruits with coarse skins
    D. angel food cake   (8:318)

61. Of the following, the food *not* generally included in a liquid diet is

    A. cooked fruit
    B. malted milk
    C. eggnog
    D. chocolate   (8:319)

62. Of the following, the food *not* generally included in a liquid diet is

    A. well strained gruels
    B. puréed vegetables
    C. ice cream
    D. Bulgarian milk   (8:319)

63. Of the following, the food *not* generally included in a liquid diet is

    A. jello
    B. soft cooked eggs
    C. clear broth
    D. rennet custard   (8:319)

64. Fluid diet may include

    A. coffee
    B. milk
    C. orange juice
    D. all of the above   (8:319)

65. Of the following, the diet which involves a modification in the consistency of the regular diet is the

    A. high caloric
    B. purine free
    C. soft
    D. salt free   (8:318)

66. Of the following foods, the one permitted in a full liquid diet but not allowed on a clear-liquid diet is

    A. milk
    B. chicken broth
    C. fruit juices
    D. tea, coffee, ginger ale (8:320)

67. A food which is included in a full liquid diet but *not* a clear-liquid diet is

    A. ice cream
    B. broth
    C. gelatin
    D. tea   (8:320)

68. Of the following, the food which may generally be included in a restricted liquid diet is

    A. strained soup with milk
    B. unstrained fruit juices
    C. cereal water
    D. buttermilk   (8:320)

69. Of the following, the food *not* generally included in a restricted liquid diet is

    A. albumin
    B. strained soup
    C. simple desserts
    D. Postum   (8:320)

70. Of the following, the food *not* generally included in a restricted liquid diet is

    A. well strained fruit juice
    B. well cooked cereal
    C. ices
    D. jello   (8:320)

71. When a patient is suffering from fever accompanied by rapid metabolism, he should generally be put on a

    A. low protein diet
    B. low fat diet
    C. high calorie diet
    D. low purine diet   (8:328)

72. As compared with the amount needed in good health, the amount of protein needed with fevers is

    A. much greater
    B. much less

C. slightly greater
D. slightly less   (8:328)

73. During the acute stage of fever, it is important to

   A. increase the allotment of cellulose
   B. increase the fluid intake
   C. "starve" the patient
   D. discontinue proteins   (8:328)

74. The normal diet is modified by increasing the caloric value in cases of

   A. arthritis
   B. diabetes mellitus
   C. cardiac diseases
   D. typhoid fever   (8:329)

75. Of the following diseases, the one *not* caused by a lack of essential food elements is

   A. rickets
   B. scurvy
   C. beriberi
   D. emphysema   (8:334)

76. The chief feature of the Meulengracht diet, often prescribed for bleeding ulcers, is

   A. high fat content
   B. puréed fruits and vegetables
   C. low protein content
   D. whole grain cereals   (8:344)

77. Most nutritional authorities agree that mineral oil does not interfere with the absorption of

   A. vitamin K
   B. vitamin D
   C. vitamin C
   D. vitamin A   (8:351)

78. The prescribed diet in chronic gastritis must be

   A. adequate in calories
   B. adequate in nutrients
   C. soft in consistency
   D. all of the above   (8:346)

79. A bland diet is usually prescribed for

   A. gastric disorders
   B. diabetes mellitus
   C. gallbladder diseases
   D. overweight   (8:346)

80. Food found in a bland diet is generally *not*

   A. stimulating
   B. nonirritating
   C. digestible
   D. nonresidue-forming   (8:346)

81. Diets based on modifications of consistency are most applicable to patients afflicted with

   A. tuberculosis
   B. deficiencies in vitamin A and C
   C. ulcers of the gastrointestinal tract or inflammation of the gastrointestinal tract
   D. allergies   (8:346)

82. A low-residue diet is used primarily for

   A. atonic constipation
   B. hyperacidity
   C. malnutrition
   D. diarrhea   (8:355)

83. The Schmidt test diet is used to determine the food which causes

   A. liver disorders
   B. kidney stones
   C. enteritis
   D. cholelithiasis   (8:359)

84. The low-fat high-carbohydrate diet is used for people suffering from diseases of the

   A. kidney
   B. heart
   C. intestines
   D. liver   (8:369)

85. An increased proportion of carbohydrate is required in the dietary treatment of

   A. diabetes mellitus
   B. gout
   C. liver disease
   D. obesity   (8:365)

86. A low-fat diet is usually prescribed for patients having

    A. diseases of the liver
    B. epilepsy
    C. tuberculosis
    D. anemia (8:369)

87. Of the following, the group which is generally excluded in a low-fat diet is

    A. gravies, butter, oil
    B. green vegetables and salad plants
    C. whole grain products and legumes
    D. fish and milk (8:370)

88. The preoperative diet should prevent acidosis by containing a high percentage of

    A. broth
    B. milk
    C. hard candy
    D. white bread (8:373)

89. A patient allowed only water, clear tea, black coffee, and clear broth is said to be on a

    A. surgical fluid diet
    B. low salt diet
    C. unrestricted fluid diet
    D. full fluid diet (8:374)

90. Of the following foods, the one believed to be the most frequent producer of allergic reactions is

    A. gelatin
    B. lamb
    C. wheat
    D. lemons (8:388)

91. Of the following, the food most likely to cause allergic reactions is

    A. lamb
    B. eggs
    C. pears
    D. peaches (8:388)

92. Food allergies are most common due to which of the following classes of foods?

    A. protein
    B. carbohydrate
    C. mineral
    D. fat (8:388)

93. Rowe elimination diets are used in cases involving

    A. allergy
    B. lead poisoning
    C. constipation
    D. nephritis (8:390)

94. The food to be omitted from a diet of a patient allergic to milk is

    A. Ry-Krisp wafers
    B. mayonnaise
    C. butter
    D. gelatin (8:391)

95. Of the following foods, the one which a patient sensitive to wheat must avoid is

    A. puffed rice
    B. milk
    C. gelatin
    D. malted milk (8:391)

96. Of the following foods, the one highest in purine is

    A. dairy products
    B. vegetables
    C. glandular organs
    D. fruits (8:420)

97. A diet which is "purine free" may contain

    A. milk and fruits
    B. milk and calves liver
    C. calves liver and bacon
    D. beefsteak and vegetables (8:420)

98. In cases of advanced gout, the purine content of the daily diet is restricted to

    A. 10 to 15 mg
    B. 50 to 60 mg
    C. 100 to 150 mg
    D. 500 to 650 mg (8:420)

99. The group of foods which is generally excluded in a low purine diet is

    A. fruit juice and milk products
    B. meats, kidney, liver
    C. eggs, fruits, nuts
    D. desserts, sugars, vegetables   (8:421)

100. Of the following modifications, the one which is most advisable for reduction in weight is

    A. reduction in fluids
    B. increase in fat
    C. reduction in calories
    D. addition of vitamins   (8:426)

101. The group of foods which contribute most to the formation of uric acid is

    A. green vegetables and citrus fruits
    B. dried fruits and whole grain cereals
    C. potatoes and eggs
    D. meat and fish   (8:420)

102. The characteristics of a reducing diet for an obese person are

    A. low in caloric value, fat, and carbohydrate; normal or high in protein, vitamins and minerals
    B. low in caloric value, fat, carbohydrate, protein, and vitamins
    C. low in caloric value, vitamins, and minerals; normal or high in carbohydrate
    D. low in caloric value and high in fat   (8:427)

103. Of the following, the food which is *not* generally allowed in treating obesity is

    A. buttermilk
    B. butter
    C. string beans
    D. soft cheese   (8:427)

104. In a reducing diet, the number of calories allowed daily depends on the

    A. weight of the patient
    B. build of the person
    C. amount of food a person eats
    D. total activity of the person   (8:427)

105. When planning a diet for an overweight adolescent girl, it is most important to consider that

    A. the chief problem is controlling the intake of candy and rich desserts
    B. excess weight often disappears by the end of the adolescent period
    C. most problems of overweight are glandular in origin
    D. emotional and social problems are often related to the obesity   (8:433)

106. A high calorie diet usually consists of the liquid part of the soft diet plus a caloric value increase through the addition of carbohydrates and fats in the form of

    A. fat meats, gravies, pastries
    B. green vegetables, meat, fish
    C. milk, sugar, cream
    D. salad greens, dried fruits, molasses   (8:436)

107. Assume that a young patient has been losing weight and that she has been given instructions for a high-calorie diet. Of the following instructions, the one which is *not* correct in this case is

    A. to be sure to eat a protein food at each meal
    B. to take a high calorie feeding between meals if this will not decrease your appetite
    C. to increase the intake of thiamine, as it will improve your appetite
    D. not to use fat in the diet because fat increases the satiety value of meals   (8:436)

108. When it is necessary to recommend a diet for the purpose of adding weight, the one which is most advisable is

    A. a low fat diet
    B. a nonroughage diet
    C. a low protein diet
    D. a high carbohydrate diet   (8:436)

109. The Karell diet is used in the care of

    A. Addison's diease

B. cardiac conditions
C. diabetes
D. jaundice   (8:440)

110. The type of diet which would most probably be recommended by the dietitian when
a patient is suffering from edema is a

A. high calorie diet
B. roughage diet
C. diet rich in mineral salts
D. low salt diet   (8:441)

111. Of the following conditions, the one cal-
ling for modification of the normal diet by
restricting sodium is

A. tuberculosis
B. diabetes
C. gastritis
D. edema   (8:441)

112. Generally excluded in a low salt diet is
food containing

A. phosphorus
B. sodium chloride
C. potassium
D. iodine   (8:441)

113. Omitted in a low salt diet is

A. baked apple with whipped cream
B. American cheese
C. olive oil
D. boiled string beans   (8:441)

114. Of the following diets, the one most suita-
ble for an overweight woman with cardiac
condition and edema is

A. low caloric, low residue, low salt
B. Sippy
C. liquid nonresidue
D. bland   (8:443)

115. Of the following, the one which should *not*
be included freely on a 500 mg sodium diet
is

A. fresh flounder
B. frozen fillet of haddock

C. fresh salmon
D. dietetic canned salmon   (8:446)

116. A rice diet is usually prescribed for patients
who

A. have high blood pressure
B. have a food allergy
C. are recovering from a gallbladder
operation
D. require a high caloric intake   (8:461)

117. Of the following disease conditions, the
one requiring restriction of fluids and salt
is

A. acute nephritis with edema
B. anemia
C. pellagra
D. peptic ulcer   (8:474)

118. Of the following fruits, those which may
be included in a high acid ash diet are

A. prunes
B. oranges
C. bananas
D. pears   (8:484)

119. Of the following groups of foods, the one
containing the largest number of alkaline-ash foods is

A. milk, sugar starch
B. milk, meat, potatoes
C. all fruits and vegetables
D. most fruits and vegetables, milk
                                        (8:484)

120. In planning an alkaline-ash diet, the foods
that should be omitted are

A. apples and peaches
B. plums and cranberries
C. almonds and chestnuts
D. raisins and carrots   (8:484)

121. Foods high in acid ash include

A. eggs
B. cereal
C. meat
D. all of the above   (8:484)

122. The ketogenic diet is

    A. very high in fat and low in carbohydrate
    B. inadequate in calories
    C. high in carbohydrate and low in fat
    D. adequate in calcium   (8:487)

123. The ketogenic diet may be used to produce acidosis in the body because it

    A. is high in fat and low in carbohydrates
    B. contains the normal amount of protein which is acid producing in the body
    C. contains a high-acid ash
    D. is high in vitamin content   (8:487)

124. The sodium-restricted diet limited to 500 mg is known as the "strict" diet. Of the following statements concerning this diet, the one which is *not* correct is that

    A. any fresh meat may be used
    B. all labels on frozen vegetables packages should be read carefully, as some salt may have been used in processing
    C. the amount of fresh, dried, or frozen fruit is not restricted
    D. baking powder biscuits are not allowed unless made with sodium-free baking powder   (8:449)

125. Of the following, the disease which is *not* directly due to a lack of specific vitamins is

    A. pellagra
    B. epilepsy
    C. rickets
    D. beriberi   (8:487)

126. Infections of the eyes, respiratory tract, and lungs are generally associated with a shortage of

    A. vitamin A
    B. vitamin D
    C. vitamin E
    D. vitamin C   (8:496)

127. Of the following, the condition which is generally a result of a deficiency or absence of vitamin A in the diet is

    A. lowered resistance to infection in the alimentary canal

    B. tooth decay
    C. night blindness
    D. diarrhea   (8:494)

128. Of the following, the condition which is *not* generally a result of a deficiency or absence of vitamin A in the diet is

    A. decalcification of the bones
    B. nerve degeneration
    C. failure of appetite and digestion
    D. sterility due to failure of ovulation   (8:496)

129. Thiamine defiency causes

    A. pellagra
    B. tetany
    C. scurvy
    D. beriberi   (8:497)

130. Beriberi is a deficiency disease caused by the lack of

    A. thiamine
    B. vitamin C
    C. vitamin A
    D. vitamin B_{12} (8:497)

131. The cure of beriberi can best be accomplished by including in the diet foods containing considerable amounts of

    A. vitamin A
    B. vitamin B
    C. vitamin D
    D. vitamin C   (8:497)

132. Of the following terms, the one which might adequately be used to characterize beriberi is

    A. neuritic
    B. hemorrhagic
    C. parasitic
    D. exophthalmic   (8:497)

133. Beriberi is associated with

    A. enlargement of the heart
    B. dropsy or edema
    C. incoordination of movements
    D. muscle weakness
    E. all of the above   (8:498)

134. Of the following, the condition which is not generally a result of a deficiency or absence of vitamin B in the diet is

   A. sterility due to cessation of oestrus cycle
   B. soft and fragile bones
   C. polyneuritis
   D. impaired growth of the young in the lactation period (8:499)

135. Experimental evidence has shown that some dietary factor is a specific in the prevention or correction of all cases of

   A. tuberculosis
   B. malnutrition
   C. pellagra
   D. constipation (8:499)

136. Loss of appetite is specifically associated with a lack of

   A. vitamin C
   B. vitamin B
   C. vitamin D
   D. vitamin E (8:499)

137. Of the following, the condition which is not generally a result of deficiency or absence of vitamin B in the diet is

   A. impairment of the digestive processes
   B. anhydremia
   C. gradual paralysis of the limbs
   D. deformities of the bones (8:499)

138. Of the following, the symptom most indicative of riboflavin deficiency is

   A. poor wound healing
   B. fissures at the corners of the mouth
   C. bone deformities
   D. simple goiter (8:499)

139. Of the following, the condition which is *not* generally a result of a deficiency or absence of vitamin C in the diet is

   A. bleeding muscles and tissues
   B. loss of weight
   C. pellagra
   D. loosening and shedding of teeth (8:499)

140. If a pregnant woman does not drink milk, the lack of calcium and riboflavin can best be compensated for by using greater amounts of

   A. fruits and yellow vegetables
   B. green and yellow vegetables
   C. hard cheese and green leafy vegetables
   D. hard cheese and butter (8:499)

141. Of the following conditions, the one which is *not* generally a result of a deficiency or absence of vitamin C in the diet is

   A. fragility of bones
   B. diarrhea
   C. scurvy
   D. sallow or pallid complexion (8:501)

142. Experimental evidence has shown that some dietary factor is specific in the prevention or correction of all cases of

   A. gastric ulcers
   B. scurvy
   C. overweight
   D. tooth decay (8:501)

143. Scurvy is a disease due to a diet inadequate in

   A. vitamin C
   B. vitamin A
   C. vitamin B
   D. vitamin D (8:501)

144. Of the following statements, the one most nearly accurate is

   A. scurvy will develop without citrus fruits
   B. vitamin C must be provided to prevent scurvy
   C. if children have signs of latent scurvy it is because they did not have orange juice
   D. orange juice is the cheapest source of vitamin C (8:501)

145. Of the following, the one which is *not* generally a result of a deficiency or absence of vitamin D in the diet is

   A. poorly calcified teeth

B. pigmentation and thickening of the skin
C. bowed legs
D. enlargement of rib junctions   (8:502)

146. Of the following, the condition which is *not* generally a result of a deficiency or absence of vitamin D in the diet is

A. general muscular weakness
B. retention and deposition of the boneforming elements, calcium and phosphorus, in the body
C. failure of placental functioning in the female
D. bulging forehead   (8:504)

147. Iodine deficiency is first manifested in the

A. liver
B. thyroid
C. teeth structure
D. veins of the neck   (8:506)

148. A possible result of protein deficiency is

A. edema
B. heart disease
C. gout
D. sprue   (8:510)

149. Lack of iodine in the diet may cause

A. simple goiter
B. scurvy
C. pellagra
D. anemia
E. tetany   (8:506)

150. In phenylketonuria, there is a disturbance in the metabolism of

A. thyroxine
B. tyrosine
C. cystine
D. valine   (8:532)

151. Hypoproteinemia may be seen in

A. chronic diarrhea
B. febrile states
C. elevated basal metabolic rate
D. all of the above   (8:510)

152. The food permitted on a diet which is wheat free, rye free, and oat free is

A. malted milk
B. rice pudding
C. canned tomato soup
D. bologna   (8:514)

153. Of the following groups of foods, the one which may be indicated in a gluten free diet is

A. rye, barley, macaroni
B. crackers, spaghetti, rice
C. cream of wheat, cornstarch, oats
D. corn, potato, rice   (8:514)

154. In the treatment of phenylketonuria, the diet must be modified so that

A. all protein is eliminated from the diet
B. phenylalanine is completely eliminated from the diet until the child is 5 years old
C. the serum level of phenylalanine is maintained within normal limits
D. milk and milk products are the only foods eliminated from the diet (8:532)

155. The protein found in milk is

A. casein
B. lactose
C. gluten
D. albumin   (8:560)

156. the most important contribution of fruit in the diet is its

A. vitamin content
B. high caloric value
C. satiety value
D. acid reaction   (8:590)

157. Which is highest in calcium content?

A. cheddar cheese
B. cheese spread
C. bread
D. beans   (8:678)

158. A diet deficient in calcium may be corrected by adding

A. buttermilk, cheese, ice cream
B. creamed toast, eggs, molasses
C. tomatoes, cheese, macaroni
D. eggs, milk, tomatoes   (8:678)

159. Of the following, the food richest in calcium is

A. oysters
B. cheese
C. celery
D. carrots   (8:678-9)

160. Which is lowest in calcium?

A. oranges
B. beet greens
C. baked custard
D. collards   (8:679)

161. Of the following foods, the poorest source of iron is

A. cabbage
B. almonds
C. cocoa
D. oysters   (8:680)

162. Of the following foods, the best source of iron is

A. asparagus
B. graham bread
C. oatmeal
D. egg yolk   (8:680)

163. Of the following foods, the best source of iron is

A. whole eggs
B. cheese
C. raisins
D. dried peas   (8:680)

164. Which of the following contains the highest amount of sodium?

A. beef
B. lamb
C. ham
D. pork   (8:682)

Answer the questions in this group by following the directions below:

A. if only A is correct
B. if only B is correct
C. if both A and B are correct
D. if both A and B are incorrect

165. Monosaccharides occurring free in foods include

A. glucose
B. fructose
C. both
D. neither   (8:41)

166. Mannitol

A. is easily digested
B. yields about one-half the calories per gram as fructose
C. both
D. neither   (8:42)

167. Fructose can be found in

A. fruit
B. honey
C. both
D. neither   (8:42)

168. Fruits contain

A. glucose
B. fructose
C. both
D. neither   (8:49)

169. Starch can be found in

A. grains
B. legumes
C. both
D. neither   (8:44)

170. Lipids important in nutrition include

A. cerebrosides
B. gangliosides
C. both
D. neither   (8:53)

171. Cholesterol can be found in

    A. egg yolk
    B. animal fat
    C. both
    D. neither   (8:58)

172. Calcium is necessary for

    A. hemoglobin formation
    B. normal thyroid gland function
    C. both
    D. neither   (8:101)

173. Minerals are essential for the formation of

    A. bones
    B. teeth
    C. both
    D. neither   (8:101)

174. Iron is found in

    A. liver
    B. egg yolk
    C. both
    D. neither   (8:107)

175. Dietary sodium restriction is indicated in

    A. cardiovascular disorders
    B. pulmonary tuberculosis
    C. both
    D. neither   (8:111)

176. Potassium is found in

    A. fruits
    B. milk
    C. both
    D. neither   (8:112)

177. Riboflavin deficiency is associated with

    A. perforation of the nasal septum
    B. depression of the sternum
    C. both
    D. neither   (8:133)

178. Pharmaceutical sources of vitamin K include

    A. wheat germ
    B. egg yolk

    C. both
    D. neither   (8:146)

179. Vitamins are necessary for the functioning of

    A. the heart
    B. the nerves
    C. both
    D. neither   (8:146)

180. The average diet of an adult includes

    A. 60 to 90 g of proteins
    B. 100 to 150 g of carbohydrates
    C. both
    D. neither   (8:309)

181. A light diet may contain

    A. fried foods
    B. coarse foods
    C. both
    D. neither   (8:316)

182. A light diet may contain

    A. orange juice
    B. milk
    C. both
    D. neither   (8:317)

183. A general diet may contain

    A. cooked asparagus
    B. macaroni and cheese
    C. both
    D. neither   (8:317)

184. The "full" diet contains

    A. 1500 calories
    B. 200 to 300 g of carbohydrates
    C. both
    D. neither   (8:316)

185. The "house" diet contains

    A. 70 g of proteins
    B. 150 g of fats
    C. both
    D. neither   (8:316)

186. In some hospitals, the general diet is known as

   A. "regular diet"
   B. "full" diet
   C. both
   D. neither   (8:316)

187. A soft diet is

   A. low in cellulose
   B. high in connective tissue
   C. both
   D. neither   (8:318)

188. High fiber diet may contain

   A. cooked green beans
   B. cooked spinach
   C. both
   D. neither   (8:352)

189. A clear liquid diet is composed chiefly of

   A. water
   B. carbohydrates
   C. both
   D. neither   (8:320)

190. Patients with gallbladder disease must avoid

   A. chocolate
   B. nuts
   C. both
   D. neither   (8:369)

191. The diet for viral hepatitis is high in

   A. protein
   B. carbohydrate
   C. both
   D. neither   (8:363)

192. Patients with gallbladder disease can eat

   A. soft fiber foods
   B. fried foods
   C. both
   D. neither   (8:369)

193. The diet for dumping syndrome includes

   A. avoidance of sugar
   B. small frequent feedings
   C. both
   D. neither   (8:379)

194. A patient sensitive to milk must avoid

   A. cheese
   B. ice cream
   C. both
   D. neither   (8:391)

195. A patient on an egg-poor diet can eat

   A. breads with glazed crusts
   B. meringues
   C. both
   D. neither   (8:391)

196. A patient on wheat poor diet can have

   A. soy bread
   B. beer
   C. both
   D. neither   (8:391)

197. Foods high in acid ash include

   A. fish
   B. bread
   C. both
   D. neither   (8:484)

198. The ketogenic diet which may be used in the treatment of epilepsy contains a

   A. high amount of carbohydrate
   B. low amount of fat
   C. both
   D. neither   (8:487)

199. Iodine deficiency in the food may cause

   A. overweight
   B. chlorosis
   C. both
   D. neither   (8:506)

200. Magnesium deficiency causes

   A. convulsions
   B. nervous irritability
   C. both
   D. neither   (8:509)

Answer Key: Nutrition and Diet Therapy

1. C	26. A	51. A	76. B	101. D	126. A	151. D	176. C
2. A	27. A	52. C	77. C	102. A	127. C	152. B	177. D
3. D	28. A	53. B	78. D	103. B	128. A	153. D	178. D
4. A	29. D	54. A	79. A	104. D	129. D	154. C	179. C
5. D	30. A	55. B	80. A	105. D	130. A	155. A	180. A
6. D	31. D	56. A	81. C	106. C	131. B	156. A	181. D
7. D	32. A	57. C	82. D	107. D	132. A	157. A	182. C
8. B	33. D	58. A	83. C	108. D	133. E	158. A	183. C
9. D	34. B	59. C	84. D	109. B	134. B	159. B	184. B
10. D	35. B	60. C	85. C	110. D	135. C	160. A	185. A
11. D	36. B	61. A	86. A	111. D	136. B	161. A	186. C
12. D	37. B	62. B	87. A	112. B	137. D	162. D	187. A
13. C	38. C	63. B	88. C	113. B	138. B	163. D	188. C
14. D	39. C	64. D	89. A	114. A	139. C	164. C	189. A
15. C	40. A	65. C	90. C	115. B	140. C	165. C	190. C
16. C	41. C	66. A	91. B	116. A	141. B	166. B	191. C
17. B	42. A	67. A	92. A	117. A	142. B	167. C	192. A
18. D	43. B	68. C	93. A	118. A	143. A	168. C	193. C
19. D	44. B	69. C	94. C	119. D	144. B	169. C	194. C
20. C	45. C	70. B	95. D	120. B	145. B	170. C	195. D
21. D	46. B	71. C	96. C	121. D	146. C	171. C	196. D
22. C	47. C	72. C	97. A	122. A	147. B	172. D	197. C
23. A	48. A	73. B	98. C	123. A	148. A	173. C	198. D
24. C	49. A	74. D	99. B	124. C	149. A	174. C	199. D
25. C	50. C	75. D	100. C	125. B	150. B	175. A	200. C

Chapter Eight

Maternal and Child Health Nursing

Directions: Select from among the lettered choices the one that most appropriately answers the question or completes the statement.

1. The most common cause of maternal death in the U.S. is

   A. hemorrhage ✓
   B. toexemia
   C. infection
   D. hypertension   (6:15)

2. Causes of maternal mortality include

   A. hemorrhage
   B. toxemia
   C. infection
   D. all of the above ✓   (6:15)

3. The zygote contains how many chromosomes?

   A. 13
   B. 23
   C. 43
   D. 46 ✓   (6:66)

4. The endometrium during pregnancy is called the

   A. decidua ✓
   B. ectoderm
   C. blastodermic vesicle
   D. trophoblast   (6:77)

5. How long after conception is the ovum implanted in the endometrium?

   A. 3 to 4 days later ✓
   B. immediately
   C. 5 hours later
   D. 24 hours later   (6:77)

6. Which of the following is not true of the amniotic fluid?

   A. its normal amount is from 700 to 2000 cc
   B. it represents a mechanical protection for the fetus
   C. it is slightly acid ✓
   D. its color is yellowish   (6:79)

7. By what month of pregnancy is the placenta formed?

   A. second
   B. third ✓
   C. fourth
   D. fifth   (6:79)

8. The placenta at term weighs

   A. 1500 g
   B. 500 to 600 g
   C. one-third of the weight of the fetus ✓
   D. 300 g   (6:81)

9. A patient expels a fetus of 6 1/2 inches prematurely. The approximate age of the fetus is

   A. 2 months
   B. 3 months
   C. 4 months
   D. 5 months ✓   (6:84)

10. By what week of gestation can the fetal heartbeat be heard?

    A. sixth
    B. ninth
    C. twelfth
    D. twentieth ✓   (6:84)

11. In what week of pregnancy do the teeth begin to form in the gums?

    A. second
    B. third
    C. fifth
    D. twelfth ✓   (6:84)

12. If a pregnant woman's last menstrual period began on June 10, the estimated due date would be near

    A. February 10
    B. February 17
    C. March 10 ✓
    D. March 17   (6:86)

13. During pregnancy how much is the uterus increased in size?

    A. 100%
    B. 200%
    C. 300%
    D. 500% ✓   (6:109)

14. The increased size of the uterus during pregnancy results from

    A. growth of new muscle fibers
    B. stretching of the muscle fibers
    C. enlargement of pre-existent muscle fibers
    D. all of the above ✓   (6:109)

15. The precursor of breast milk, colostrum, can first be expressed in the

    A. first trimester
    B. second trimester
    C. third trimester
    D. postpartum period ✓   (6:115)

16. At the end of the first trimester of pregnancy, there is

    A. an increase in blood volume ✓
    B. a decrease in the stroke volume of the heart
    C. an increase in diastolic blood pressure
    D. all of the above   (6:115)

17. During the first trimester of pregnancy the weight gain is

    A. 5 lbs ✓
    B. 8 lbs
    C. 12 lbs
    D. none of the above   (6:115)

18. The major endocrine gland involved in pregnancy is the

    A. thyroid
    B. placenta ✓
    C. adrenal
    D. pituitary   (6:118)

19. Probable signs of pregnancy include

    A. enlargement of the abdomen
    B. fetal outline distinguished by abdominal palpation
    C. Hegar's sign
    D. all of the above ✓   (6:119)

20. Danger signals during pregnancy include

    A. pain in the abdomen
    B. chills and fever
    C. sudden escape of fluid from the vagina
    D. all of the above ✓   (6:133)

21. How many grams of protein does the average woman need daily?

    A. 30
    B. 45 ✓
    C. 60
    D. 75   (6:140)

22. During which period of pregnancy does the fetus store the greatest amounts of iron?

    A. first trimester
    B. second trimester
    C. third trimester ✓
    D. the storage is equal in every trimester (6:147)

23. Minor discomforts of pregnancy include

    A. nausea
    B. heartburn
    C. varicose veins
    D. all of the above   (6:162,163)

24. A pregnant patient has painful, distended veins in the legs. This condition is most likely due to

    A. pressure against the veins in the pelvis
    B. infection of the veins
    C. pressure against the abdominal aorta
    D. all of the above   (6:162,163)

25. In a primipara, the average length of labor is

    A. 4 to 6 hours
    B. 6 to 8 hours
    C. 8 to 11 hours
    D. 12 to 18 hours   (6:217)

26. Following delivery of the placenta, methergine is given in order to

    A. relax the uterus
    B. stimulate uterine contractions
    C. increase lactation
    D. suppress lactation   (6:271)

27. The puerperium period usually lasts

    A. 2 to 3 weeks
    B. 3 to 5 weeks
    C. 5 to 8 weeks
    D. 6 to 12 weeks   (6:293)

28. On the third day of the puerperium, the lochia are expected to be

    A. lochia rubra
    B. lochia alba
    C. lochia serosa
    D. none of the above   (6:294)

29. Preeclampsia is characterized by

    A. elevation in blood pressure
    B. albuminuria
    C. edema
    D. all of the above   (6:449)

30. Danger signals during pregnancy include

    A. swelling of the face and fingers
    B. vaginal bleeding
    C. persistent vomiting
    D. all of the above   (6:448,458)

31. A patient with mild preeclampsia receives chlorothiazide therapy. She should be advised to take chlorothiazide together with

    A. orange juice
    B. penicillin
    C. aspirin
    D. vitamin A   (6:452)

32. Magnesium sulfate is given to eclamptic patients in order to achieve

    A. increased diuresis
    B. control of convulsions
    C. peripheral vasodilatation
    D. all of the above   (6:455)

33. Which of the following is an unfavorable sign in a patient with eclampsia

    A. a sustained pulse rate over 120
    B. temperature over 103°F
    C. 10 or more g of albumin per liter of urine
    D. all of the above   (6:454)

34. The most common drug used in eclamptic patients is

    A. morphine
    B. codeine
    C. chloral hydrate
    D. magnesium sulfate   (6(455)

35. Maternal mortality with modern management of eclampsia is

    A. 85 to 90%
    B. about 60%
    C. 20 to 25%
    D. less than 10%   (6:454)

36. Therapeutic abortion is indicated when the patient has

    A. tuberculosis
    B. diabetes

C. influenza
D. none of the above ✓ (6:459)

37. A patient in early pregnancy has some vaginal bleeding and mild cramps, but the cervix is closed. This patient probably has

A. missed abortion
B. threatened abortion ✓
C. incomplete abortion
D. none of the above (6:459)

38. A self-induced abortion is called

A. ectopic
B. habitual
C. criminal ✓
D. missed abortion (6:460)

39. When the placenta is attached to the lower uterine segment, it is called

A. placenta previa ✓
B. placenta abruptio
C. placenta circumvalata
D. placenta membranacea (6:466)

40. Treatment of hyperemesis gravidarum includes administration of

A. parenteral fluids
B. thiamine chloride
C. sedatives
D. all of the above ✓ (6:469)

41. Syphilis in a pregnant woman is treated with

A. arsenicals
B. penicillin ✓
C. tetracycline
D. bismuth (6:474)

42. Cessation of progress in labor because of abnormalities in the mechanics involved is called

A. dysfunction
B. dystocia ✓
C. hypertonia
D. effacement (6(476)

43. Treatment for hypertonic uterine dysfunction includes

A. rest
B. fluids
C. morphine
D. all of the above ✓ (6:478)

44. Facial paralysis of the baby seen right after delivery is usually associated with

A. congenital syphilis
B. spina bifida
C. forceps delivery
D. hydrocephalus (6:542)

45. Pathology in an Rh positive baby born to an Rh negative mother includes

A. hydrops fetalis
B. erythroblastosis fetalis
C. anemia
D. all of the above ✓ (6:557)

46. If the newborn baby requires an exchange transfusion, it will receive

A. Rh negative blood ✓
B. Rh positive blood
C. plasma
D. O positive blood (6:559)

47. Who discovered the means of transmission of puerperal fever?

A. Meigs
B. Hodge
C. Oliver Wendell Holmes and Ignaz Semmelweis ✓
D. Kalletschka (6:598)

48. The white, cheesy matter covering the skin of the newborn infant is called

A. smegma
B. lanugo
C. vernix ✓
D. vertex (6:622)

Answer the questions in this group by following the directions below. Select

A. if only A is correct
B. if only B is correct
C. if both A and B are correct
D. if both A and B are incorrect

49. A decrease in maternal deaths during the past half century has been achieved by reducing the incidence of

   A. toxemia of pregnancy
   B. puerperal infection
   C. both ✓
   D. neither   (6:15)

50. Each spermatozoon contains

   A. 22 regular chromosomes
   B. an X or a Y chromosome
   C. both ✓
   D. neither   (6:75)

51. Each mature ovum contains

   A. 24 regular chromosomes
   B. an X chromosome ✓
   C. both ✓
   D. neither   (6:75)

52. The amniotic fluid

   A. is secreted by the placenta
   B. keeps the embryo warm and moist
   C. both ✓
   D. neither   (6:79)

53. The inferior vena cava in the fetus brings

   A. venous blood from the body
   B. arterial blood from the placenta
   C. both ✓
   D. neither   (6:89)

54. Fetal structures obliterated after birth include

   A. ductus arteriosus ✓
   B. inferior vena cava
   C. both
   D. neither   (6:89)

55. The lungs of the fetus contain

   A. air
   B. blood ✓
   C. both
   D. neither   (6:89)

56. The placenta acts as an organ

   A. providing nourishment to the fetus
   B. of gaseous exchange between mother and fetus
   C. both ✓
   D. neither   (6:89)

57. The location of the fetal heart sounds as heard through the stethoscope, gives information about

   A. fetal position ✓
   B. the sex of the fetus
   C. both
   D. neither   (6:101)

58. During pregnancy the

   A. level of fasting blood sugar is higher
   B. secretion of insulin by the pancreas is decreased
   C. both ✓
   D. neither   (6:115)

59. During pregnancy there is

   A. an increased production of red blood cells by the bone marrow ✓
   B. a decreased demand for iron
   C. both
   D. neither   (6:115)

60. Minimal hematologic values for a pregnant woman are

   A. hemoglobin 9 g ✓
   B. hematocrit 25% ✓
   C. both
   D. neither   (6:115)

61. Signs that a pregnant patient may notice in the first trimester of pregnancy include enlargement of the

   A. uterus
   B. breasts ✓
   C. both
   D. neither   (6:114)

62. Presumptive signs of pregnancy include

   A. "morning sickness" ✓
   B. "quickening" ✓
   C. both
   D. neither   (6:119)

63. "Morning sickness" usually

    A. occurs in the early part of the day ✓
    B. occurs about 8 weeks after the first menstrual period is missed
    C. both
    D. neither   (6:120)

64. The Braxton-Hicks sign is

    A. a positive sign of pregnancy
    B. perceptible in the early weeks of preg- ✓ nancy
    C. both
    D. neither   (6:122)

65. Pregnancy can be diagnosed by the

    A. Friedman test
    B. Aschheim-Zondek test
    C. both ✓
    D. neither   (6:123)

66. A woman in the eighth week of gestation will show

    A. the fetal skeleton on x-rays
    B. "quickening"
    C. both
    D. neither ✓   (6:125)

67. Laboratory tests carried out during antepartal care include

    A. urinalysis for albumin
    B. urinalysis for sugar
    C. both ✓
    D. neither   (6:130)

68. The pregnant woman is advised to have a quart of milk in her daily diet unless she develops

    A. constipation
    B. rapid weight gain
    C. both
    D. neither ✓   (6:144)

69. Daily care of the breasts during pregnancy includes

    A. daily washing ✓
    B. application of iodine
    C. both
    D. neither   (6:155)

70. A pregnant woman has flat nipples on both breasts. In preparation for breast feeding, this can be corrected by

    A. use of suction cups applied on both breasts
    B. pressing the nipples between the thumb and forefinger and rolling them gently
    C. both
    D. neither   (6:155)

71. A physician should be consulted immediately if a pregnant woman develops

    A. morning nausea
    B. constipation
    C. both
    D. neither   (6:160)

72. Heartburn during pregnancy results from

    A. increased stomach acidity
    B. reverse peristalsis causing regurgitation of the stomach contents into the esophagus
    C. both
    D. neither   (6:161)

73. Nausea and vomiting in early pregnancy may be related to

    A. slowing of peristalsis
    B. change in hormonal balance
    C. both
    D. neither   (6:160)

74. Nausea and vomiting in early pregnancy may be relieved by

    A. eating dry toast before getting out of bed
    B. taking small meals high in carbohydrates
    C. both
    D. neither   (6:160)

75. Varicose veins in pregnancy may be relieved by

A. abandonment of round garters
B. use of elastic stockings
C. both
D. neither   (6:163)

76. Leg cramps during pregnancy have been at-
tributed to

A. insufficient calcium in the diet
B. tense body posture
C. both
D. neither   (6:165)

77. Symptoms of approaching labor include

A. desire to bear down
B. appearance of "show"
C. both
D. neither   (6:213)

78. The actual onset of labor is marked by the

A. rupture of the bag of waters
B. regular contractions of the uterus
C. both
D. neither   (6:215)

79. In a primipara, the average length of labor is

A. 2 hours in the second stage
B. 30 minutes in the third stage
C. both
D. neither   (6:217)

80. In a multipara, the average length of labor is

A. 10 hours in the first stage
B. 2 hours in the second stage
C. both
D. neither   (6:217)

81. Effacement of the cervix during labor is also
called

A. "obliteration" of the cervix
B. "taking up" of the cervix
C. both
D. neither   (6:219)

82. The third stage of labor

A. begins with the delivery of the baby

B. ends with the birth of the placenta
C. both
D. neither   (6:218)

83. The second stage of labor

A. is called the placental stage
B. ends with the delivery of the baby
C. both
D. neither   (6:218)

84. The first stage of labor

A. begins with the first true labor contrac-
tion
B. ends with the complete dilatation of the
cervix
C. both
D. neither   (6:218)

85. During the second stage of labor, the contractions are

A. strong
B. long
C. both
D. neither   (6:220)

86. The contractions of the second stage of labor

A. last 10 to 15 seconds
B. occur at intervals of 10 to 12 minutes
C. both
D. neither   (6:220)

87. Precipitate labor may result from

A. very strong uterine contractions
B. abnormally low resistance of the soft
parts of the pelvis
C. both
D. neither   (6:279)

88. The period of the puerperium includes

A. progressive changes in the breasts for
lactation
B. involution of the internal reproductive
organs
C. both
D. neither   (6:293)

89. Eclampsia is characterized by

    A. convulsions
    B. coma
    C. both
    D. neither   (6:449)

90. Preeclampsia is

    A. a disease of the first 2 or 3 months of pregnancy
    B. particularly prone to occur in young primigravidae
    C. both
    D. neither   (6:449)

91. A physician should be consulted immediately if a pregnant patient has

    A. sudden excessive weight gain
    B. severe continuous headache
    C. both
    D. neither   (6:450)

92. A patient with preeclampsia receives hydrochlorothiazide. This medication will

    A. remove sodium and potassium from the body
    B. depress the appetite
    C. both
    D. neither   (6:451)

93. Early symptoms of preeclampsia may include

    A. muscular twitchings
    B. torpor
    C. both
    D. neither   (6:452)

94. Occurrence of eclampsia is higher in

    A. twin gestations
    B. primigravidae
    C. both
    D. neither   (6:454)

95. Rapid-acting barbiturates are often used in patients with eclampsia because they

    A. lower the blood pressure
    B. control convulsions
    C. both
    D. neither   (6:455)

96. Eclampsia

    A. is a chronic disease of pregnancy
    B. has an excellent prognosis
    C. both
    D. neither   (6:454)

97. Unfavorable signs in a patient with eclampsia include

    A. edema of the lungs
    B. systolic blood pressure of over 200 mm hg
    C. both
    D. neither   (6:454)

98. An eclamptic patient receives 20% hypertonic glucose solution to achieve

    A. increased diuresis
    B. depression of the central nervous system
    C. both
    D. neither   (6:456)

99. hemorrhage in the first half of pregnancy can be caused by

    A. abortion
    B. placenta previa
    C. both
    D. neither   (6:458)

100. A woman with severe infection complicating abortion is subject to

    A. bacterial shock
    B. kidney failure
    C. both
    D. neither   (6:460)

101. An abortion may be complicated by

    A. infection
    B. hemorrhage
    C. both
    D. neither   (6:460)

102. A woman with tuberculosis who becomes pregnant requires

    A. therapeutic abortion

B. antituberculosis drug therapy
C. both
D. neither   (6:473)

103. In hypertonic uterine dysfunction, the contractions

A. are inadequate, but painful
B. occur in the latent phase of labor
C. both
D. neither   (6:477)

104. In hypotonic uterine dysfunction, the contractions

A. are inadequate
B. occur in the active phase of labor
C. both
D. neither   (6:478)

105. The appearance of the cord after the rupture of the membranes indicates

A. prolapse of the cord
B. torsion of the cord
C. both
D. neither   (6:490)

106. Babies born to diabetic mothers have a tendency towards

A. icterus
B. high birth weight
C. both
D. neither   (6:525)

107. Facial paralysis of the baby seen right after delivery requires

A. vitamin C injections
B. application of warm compresses
C. both
D. neither   (6:542)

Each statement is followed by four suggested answers. Answer according to the following key:

A. **if 1, 2, and 3 are correct**
B. **if 1 and 3 are correct**
C. **if 2 and 4 are correct**
D. **if only 4 is correct**
E. **if all are correct**

108. In order to measure the diagonal conjugate (pelvic measurement), the doctor needs

1. rubber gloves
2. a pelvimeter
3. a ruler
4. a stethoscope   (6:39)

109. The umbilical cord contains

1. the umbilical arteries
2. the umbilical vein
3. Wharton's jelly
4. the umbilical lymphatic duct   (6:83)

110. At the end of the third lunar month, the fetus

1. measures about 3 inches
2. has a distinguishable sex
3. has centers of ossification
4. weighs about 3 ounces   (6:83)

111. Fetal structures obliterated after birth include

1. umbilical vein
2. umbilical arteries
3. ductus venosus
4. pulmonary arteries   (6:89)

112. Diagnosis of the fetal position during pregnancy can be made by

1. abdominal palpation
2. vaginal examination
3. rectal examination
4. x-rays   (6:98,99)

113. Physical findings considered abnormal in a pregnant patient include

1. increased size of the uterus
2. increased diameter of the areola of the breast
3. enlargement of the abdomen
4. enlargement of the thyroid gland
                                     (6:114,115)

114. Presumptive signs of pregnancy include

1. fetal skeleton seen by x-rays

2. menstrual suppression
3. positive pregnancy test
4. frequency of micturition   (6:119)

115. Positive signs of pregnancy include

1. fetal heart sounds heard
2. ballottement
3. fetal movements felt by the examiner
4. softening of the cervix   (6:123)

116. Substances giving positive reaction to the A-Z pregnancy test include

1. progesterone
2. estrogen
3. prolactin
4. chorionic gonadotropin   (6:123)

117. Laboratory tests carried out in antepartal care include

1. determination of blood type
2. determination of Rh factor
3. blood test for syphilis
4. determination of hemoglobin   (6:130)

118. In order to prevent anemia during pregnancy, it is important that the diet contain

1. iron
2. vitamin C
3. protein
4. fat   (6:147)

119. Forbidden activities during pregnancy include

1. sexual intercourse
2. traveling
3. tub baths
4. douching with hund-bulb syringe
       (6:158)

120. Heartburn during pregnancy may be relieved by

1. increasing intake of carbohydrates
2. decreasing intake of fats
3. decreasing intake of protein
4. use of aluminum hydroxide gel (6:161)

121. Mild cases of constipation during pregnancy may be relieved by giving

1. fluids
2. vegetables
3. coarse foods
4. dark breads   (6:162)

122. Early symptoms of preeclampsia may include

1. persistent headache
2. blurred vision
3. spots of light before the eyes
4. epigastric pain   (6:452)

123. Bleeding during pregnancy can be caused by

1. hydatidiform mole
2. placenta previa
3. abruptio placentae
4. ectopic pregnancy   (6:458)

124. The treatment for threatened abortion includes

1. penicillin
2. bed rest
3. quinine
4. administration of estrogen   (6:460)

125. Treatment of hypotonic uterine dysfunction includes

1. sponge baths
2. intravenous fluids
3. rupturing the membranes
4. administration of oxytocin   (6:478)

126. Factors predisposing to postpartal hemorrhage include

1. large size of the infant
2. twin pregnancy
3. hydramnios
4. internal podalic version   (6:486)

127. Clinical characteristics of amniotic fluid embolism include

1. cyanosis
2. sudden dyspnea

3. pulmonary edema
4. uterine contraction (6:489)

Directions: Each group of numbered words and statements is followed by the same number of lettered words, phrases or statements. For each numbered word or statement, choose the lettered item that is most closely related to it.

Questions 128 to 133
128. Primigravida F
129. Primipara C
130. Gravida A
131. Multipara D
132. Para I B
133. Para II E

    A. A pregnant woman
    B. A primipara
    C. A woman who has given birth to her first child
    D. A woman who has had two or more children
    E. A woman who has had two children
    F. A woman pregnant for the first time (6:114)

Questions 134 to 138
134. Missed abortion D
135. Incomplete abortion A
136. Therapeutic abortion B
137. Threatened abortion E
138. Spontaneous abortion C

    A. Some of the products of conception remain in the uterus
    B. Performed for medical reasons
    C. Abortion that occurs without a cause
    D. The fetus dies but is not expelled
    E. A condition indicating that an abortion may occur (6:459,460)

Questions 139 to 142
139. Antenatal C
140. Antepartal B
141. Allantois D
142. Amnion A

    A. The most internal of the fetal membranes
    B. Before labor and delivery
    C. Occurring before birth

    D. A tubular diverticulum of the posterior part of the yolk sac of the embryo (6:615)

Questions 143 to 146
143. Chloasma uterinum D
144. Chorion A
145. Colporrhaphy B
146. Cotyledon C

    A. The outermost membrane of the fertilized ovum
    B. The operation of suturing the vagina
    C. Any one of the subdivisions of the uterine surface of the placenta
    D. A cutaneous affection occurring during pregnancy (6:616-17)

Questions 147 to 150
147. Dystocia D
148. Ectopic gestation B
149. Effacement C
150. Involution A

    A. The return of the uterus to its normal condition after delivery
    B. Pregnancy in which the fetus is out of its normal place
    C. In obstetrics, the thinning and shortening of the cervix
    D. Difficult, slow, or painful birth or delivery (6:617,619)

Questions 151 to 155
151. Lanugo C
152. Lochia E
153. Secundine A
154. Show B
155. Vernix Caseosa D

    A. The placenta and membranes expelled after the birth of a child
    B. The blood-tinged mucus discharged from the vagina before or during labor
    C. The fine hair of the body of the fetus
    D. Fatty matter which covers the skin of the fetus
    E. The discharge from the genital canal during several days after delivery (6:619,622)

Directions: Select from among the lettered choices the one that most appropriately answers the question or completes the statement.

156. Neonatal death is the death of an infant in the first

    A. 4 months of life
    B. 4 weeks of life
    C. 4 days of life
    D. 4 hours of life   (7:33)

157. A stillborn infant has

    A. no heartbeat
    B. no respiration
    C. no muscular activity
    D. all of the above   (7:33)

158. Infant death is the death of a child within the first

    A. week of life
    B. two weeks of life
    C. month of life
    D. year of life   (7:33)

159. Fetal death is the death of a baby weighing

    A. 100 grams or more
    B. 300 grams or more
    C. 500 grams or more
    D. 1200 grams or more   (7:33)

160. Maternal mortality rate is the number of mothers who die per how many live births?

    A. 100
    B. 1,000
    C. 10,000
    D. 100,000   (7:33)

161. The most frequent cause of death in infants is

    A. cystic fibrosis
    B. pneumonia
    C. pyloric stenosis
    D. prematurity   (7:35)

162. The preferred site for injections in infants is the

    A. buttock
    B. lateral aspect of the midanterior thigh
    C. interior aspect of the thigh
    D. abdomen   (7:73)

163. Methods for computing medication doses for children include

    A. Fried's rule
    B. Clark's rule
    C. Young's rule
    D. all of the above   (7:72)

164. At birth, approximately how much of body weight is water?

    A. 40%
    B. 55%
    C. 77%
    D. 91%   (7:75)

165. Body water containing electrolytes is situated in the

    A. cells
    B. spaces between the cells
    C. plasma
    D. all of the above   (7:75)

166. How much of the volume of body water in the infant is intracellular?

    A. 20%
    B. 40%
    C. 50%
    D. 80%   (7:75)

167. How much of an infant's body weight is due to interstitial fluid?

    A. 10%
    B. 25%
    C. 40%
    D. 75%   (7:75)

168. Intracellular fluid in the infant accounts for about how much of body weight?

    A. 12%
    B. 25%
    C. 45%
    D. 60%   (7:75)

169. Intravenous therapy in children may be used for

    A. correction of electrolyte imbalance
    B. administration of medication
    C. feeding, when oral feeding is contraindicated
    D. all of the above   (7:76)

170. At what week of fetal life does the heart begin to beat?

    A. third
    B. fourth
    C. sixth
    D. tenth   (7:95)

171. Organogenesis of the fetus commences shortly after conception and is nearly complete at the end of the which prenatal month?

    A. second
    B. third
    C. fourth
    D. fifth   (7:95)

172. Immediately after birth, the newborn infant will be held head down to allow drainage from his pharynx of

    A. amniotic fluid
    B. blood
    C. gastric fluid
    D. all of the above   (7:99)

173. The eyes of the newborn must be treated prophylactically against

    A. trachoma
    B. gonorrheal infection
    C. diphtheria
    D. syphilis   (7:101)

174. How long after the infant's birth should the Apgar scoring chart be established?

    A. sixty seconds
    B. fifteen minutes
    C. six hours
    D. one week   (7:100)

175. Normal blood pressure in the new born at birth is about

    A. 60/40
    B. 80/46
    C. 100/75
    D. 125/86   (7:103)

176. The breathing rate of the healthy newborn infant is between

    A. 5 and 10/min
    B. 10 and 20/min
    C. 20 and 30/min
    D. 30 and 80/min   (7:103)

177. After birth, the infant has no further need of the

    A. ductus arteriosus
    B. foramen ovale
    C. ductus venosus
    D. all of the above   (7:103)

178. The posterior fontanel disappears after birth in

    A. 5 to 10 days
    B. 10 to 20 days
    C. 4 to 6 weeks
    D. 8 to 10 months   (7:104)

179. Prophylactic treatment of the eyes of the newborn against ophthalmia can be achieved with

    A. Neo-Synephrine
    B. cortisone
    C. silver nitrate
    D. pilocarpine   (7:101)

180. The suckled newborn infant is able to digest milk

    A. protein
    B. fat
    C. carbohydrate
    D. all of the above   (7:104)

181. Immediately after birth, the infant's temperature drops to about

    A. 94°F
    B. 95°F
    C. 96°F
    D. 97°F   (7:104)

182. The Moro reflex or startle reflex of the newborn disappears after

    A. 4 to 6 months
    B. 2 to 4 months
    C. 5 to 6 weeks
    D. 5 to 10 days   (7:106)

182. The newborn infant can

    A. stretch
    B. blink
    C. suck his thumb
    D. all of the above   (7:106)

184. The average length of a newborn infant (in the United States) is

    A. 30 inches
    B. 26 inches
    C. 21 inches
    D. 16 inches   (7:106)

185. The average weight of a newborn infant (in the United States) is

    A. 5 lbs
    B. 6 1/2 lbs
    C. 7 1/2 lbs
    D. 9 lbs   (7:106)

186. The length of stay in a hospital for a healthy newborn infant is

    A. 24 hours
    B. 3 days
    C. 6 days
    D. 3 weeks   (7:113)

187. A normal newborn baby sleeps approximately how many hours a day?

    A. 8
    B. 10 to 12
    C. 12 to 13
    D. 16 to 20
    E. 5 to 6   (7:119)

188. How many ounces of nourishment does the average infant consume in the first weeks of life in one feeding?

    A. 1/2 to 1
    B. 2 to 3
    C. 3 to 6
    D. 5 to 9   (7:118)

189. Formulas for full-term babies provide how many calories per ounce?

    A. 20
    B. 30

    C. 40
    D. 55   (7:118)

190. An infant can be fed

    A. evaporated milk
    B. whole milk
    C. dried milk
    D. all of the above   (7:118)

191. The premature baby has

    A. thin extremities
    B. little muscle
    C. wrinkled skin
    D. all of the above   (7:124)

192. The respirations of the premature infant are

    A. shallow
    B. rapid
    C. irregular
    D. all of the above   (7:126)

193. The common formula for premature infants has how many calories per ounce?

    A. 5
    B. 8
    C. 13
    D. 28   (7:129)

194. The oxygen concentration used for premature infants should not exceed

    A. 20%
    B. 40%
    C. 55%
    D. 75%   (7:129)

195. Hyperbilirubinemia is prevented in the premature infant with intramuscular

    A. phenobarbital
    B. vitamin C
    C. penicillin
    D. iron   (7:130)

196. Conditions associated with the birth of premature babies include

    A. incompetent uteral os
    B. placental insufficiency

C. poor maternal nutrition during pregnancy

D. all of the above   (7:132)

197. The pediatrician should be notified if an infant has

 A. bile-stained emesis
 B. distended abdomen
 C. an absence of stools
 D. all of the above   (7:140)

198. Meconium ileus is the presenting manifestation in many infants with

 A. fibrocystic disease
 B. omphalocele
 C. diaphragmatic hernia
 D. esophageal atresia   (7:140)

199. Epidemic rubella contracted in the second trimester of pregnancy may cause

 A. stillbirth
 B. an eye deformity in the infant
 C. the infant to have a low birth weight
 D. all of the above   (7:153)

200. The rubella virus, acting on the fetus during the first trimester of pregnancy, can cause

 A. microcephaly
 B. deafness
 C. heart disease
 D. all of the above   (7:153)

201. In a difficult delivery, the infant is most subject to fracture of the

 A. clavicle
 B. humerus
 C. ulna
 D. femur   (7:163)

202. Possible brain damage in the newborn is indicated by

 A. cyanosis
 B. loss of Moro reflex
 C. convulsions
 D. all of the above   (7:163)

203. Nursing care following surgery for congenital clubfoot includes

 A. elevation of the affected leg
 B. observation of the cast for signs of bleeding
 C. observation of the circulation and temperature of the toes
 D. all of the above   (7:166)

204. How long does it take for the infant to double his birth weight?

 A. 3 to 4 months
 B. 5 to 6 months
 C. 6 to 8 months
 D. 9 to 12 months   (7:171)

205. The weekly weight gain of the newborn is

 A. 3 oz
 B. 5 to 6 oz
 C. 6 to 8 oz
 D. 9 to 12 oz   (7:171)

206. How many inches does a baby add to his height in the six months after birth?

 A. 2 to 3
 B. 5 to 6
 C. 8 to 9
 D. 12 to 15   (7:171)

207. The head of a newborn measures about how many inches in circumference?

 A. 6
 B. 8
 C. 10
 D. 13   (7:172)

208. A two-year-old child usually weighs how many times his birth weight?

 A. 2
 B. 3
 C. 4
 D. 5   (7:172)

209. The first deciduous teeth to erupt in the baby are the

 A. lower central incisors

B. lower lateral incisors
C. first molars
D. second molars   (7:174)

210. During the first year of life, the infant requires daily

    A. 1500 I.U. of vitamin A
    B. 5 to 7 mg of iron
    C. 0.5 mg of thiamine
    D. all of the above   (7:183)

211. Vaccination of infants for measles may be given initially at

    A. 2 months
    B. 4 months
    C. 6 months
    D. 12 months   (7:184)

212. How soon after birth should infants be vaccinated for poliomyelitis?

    A. 2 months
    B. 1 week
    C. 1 year
    D. 2 years   (7:184)

213. Immunization of infants against diphtheria, tetanus, and pertussis may be started at

    A. 3 weeks
    B. 6 weeks
    C. 2 to 3 months
    D. 6 to 9 months   (7:184)

214. On babies operated for pyloric stenosis feedings are usually started

    A. 2 hours postoperatively
    B. 6 hours postoperatively
    C. 12 hours postoperatively
    D. 48 hours postoperatively   (7:214)

215. The most common form of pneumonia among infants is caused by

    A. pneumococcus
    B. staphylococcus
    C. streptococcus
    D. hemophilus influenzae   (7:233)

216. Purulent meningitis in infancy can be caused by

    A. meningococcus
    B. hemophilus influenzae
    C. tubercle bacillus
    D. all of the above   (7:237)

217. First degree burns are associated with

    A. erythema
    B. edema
    C. pain
    D. all of the above   (7:286)

Answer the questions in this group by following the directions below. Select

    A. if only A is correct
    B. if only B is correct
    C. if both A and B are correct
    D. if both A and B are incorrect

218. Frequent causes of death among infants include

    A. birth injuries
    B. respiratory disorders
    C. both
    D. neither   (7:36)

219. A child who has failed to grow properly may be tested for

    A. celiac disease
    B. fibrocystic disease
    C. both
    D. neither   (7:46)

220. Improperly placed injections in the child's buttocks may cause injury of the

    A. sciatic nerve
    B. brachial plexus
    C. both
    D. neither   (7:73)

221. Dehydration in the child may result from

    A. severe diarrhea
    B. extensive burns
    C. both
    D. neither   (7:75)

222. Retention of fluid in the child may occur through

A. impaired metabolism
B. impaired kidney action
C. both
D. neither   (7:75)

223. The infant becomes dehydrated much more quickly than the adult because of

A. rapid metabolic activity
B. a larger ratio of skin surface area to body fluid volume
C. both
D. neither   (7:75)

224. Parenteral fluids may be given

A. intravenously
B. orally
C. both
D. neither   (7:77)

225. Fluids may be given to the child by

A. oral administration
B. intravenous administration
C. both
D. neither   (7:76)

226. Fluid therapy may be needed for

A. replacement of abnormal losses
B. maintenance of normal fluid balance
C. both
D. neither   (7:76)

227. Infant deformity is sometimes due to

A. maternal infection with rubella
B. maternal use of thalidomide
C. both
D. neither   (7:95)

228. By the end of the fourth month of fetal life, the fetus has

A. vocal response
B. functional respiration
C. both
D. neither   (7:95)

229. Nicotine used by pregnant women has been found to cause

A. stimulation of the fetal blood pressure

B. depression of the fetal heart rate
C. both
D. neither   (7:96)

230. Nicotine used by a pregnant woman can be a contributing cause of

A. prematurity
B. high birth weight
C. both
D. neither   (7:96)

231. Irradiation of the abdomen of a pregnant woman may cause

A. arrest of embryonic development
B. malformations of the fetus
C. both
D. neither   (7:96)

232. An infant with an Apgar scoring chart under 5 needs

A. prompt diagnosis
B. treatment
C. both
D. neither   (7:100)

233. Blood pressure in the newborn is

A. easy to measure
B. characteristically high
C. both
D. neither   (7:103)

234. Breathing in the healthy newborn is

A. quiet
B. deep
C. both
D. neither   (7:103)

235. Respirations of the newborn are

A. abdominal
B. diaphragmatic
C. both
D. neither   (7:103)

236. In the newborn the

A. breasts may be enlarged due to maternal estrogens in the bloodstream

B. chest has a greater circumference than the head
C. both
D. neither   (7:104)

237. In the newborn female, the labia are prominent due to

   A. compression of the cord during delivery
   B. effects of the mother's estrogens
   C. both
   D. neither   (7:104)

238. Reflexes present before birth in the fetus include

   A. sucking reflex
   B. swallowing reflex
   C. both
   D. neither   (7:104)

239. Meconium contains

   A. fat
   B. intestinal secretions
   C. both
   D. neither   (7:104)

240. Injury to the periosteum of the skull bones is seen in

   A. caput succedaneum
   B. cephalhematoma
   C. both
   D. neither   (7:105)

241. Maternal hormones may be responsible for which of the following in a baby?

   A. vaginal bleeding
   B. prominent labia
   C. both
   D. neither   (7:104)

242. Reflexes present in the newborn infant include

   A. the rooting reflex
   B. the grasp reflex
   C. both
   D. neither   (7:107)

243. The newborn infant can

   A. swallow
   B. cough
   C. both
   D. neither   (7:106)

244. Advantages of breast milk include

   A. easy digestability
   B. no preparation requirements
   C. both
   D. neither   (7:115)

245. An infant may be unable to breast feed because of

   A. prematurity
   B. cleft lip defect
   C. both
   D. neither   (7:115)

246. Breast feeding of the newborn is contraindicated in case of maternal

   A. tuberculosis
   B. malnutrition
   C. both
   D. neither   (7:115)

247. Premature infants

   A. weigh more than 6 pounds
   B. are more than 18 inches long
   C. both
   D. neither   (7:123)

248. Premature infants have

   A. large fontanels
   B. wrinkled skin
   C. both
   D. neither   (7:124)

249. The premature infant has an

   A. underdeveloped gagging reflex
   B. overdeveloped gagging reflex
   C. both
   D. neither   (7:125)

250. Physiological handicaps of the premature infant include

A. increased shivering
B. difficult temperature control
C. both
D. neither   (7:124)

251. The premature baby has a

    A. large head compared to his body
    B. thick skin
    C. both
    D. neither   (7:124)

252. Premature infants often have

    A. relatively large fontanels
    B. a subnormal body temperature
    C. both
    D. neither   (7:125)

253. Measures to be observed in caring for a premature infant include

    A. maintenance of body temperature
    B. adequate fluid and caloric intake
    C. both
    D. neither   (7:128)

254. Premature babies are usually discharged from the hospital when they achieve a

    A. weight of 5 to 5 1/2 lbs
    B. steady weight gain
    C. both
    D. neither   (7:131)

255. Jaundice is common in prematures. In order to prevent bilirubin from reaching dangerous levels, it is common to expose babies to

    A. "blue" fluorescent lights
    B. high oxygen concentration
    C. both
    D. neither   (7:130)

256. Conditions associated with birth of premature babies include

    A. placenta abruptio
    B. diverticulosis
    C. both
    D. neither   (7:132)

257. A baby had a cleft lip repair. In the postoperative period, in order to prevent strain on the sutures, the baby should be fed with a

    A. rubber tipped asepto syringe
    B. baby spoon
    C. both
    D. neither   (7:135)

258. Tracheoesophageal fistula is often diagnosed in the newborn when the nurse notices

    A. excessive drooling
    B. cyanosis when feeding is attempted
    C. both
    D. neither   (7:136)

259. If a nurse sees an infant gagging on mucus and becoming cyanotic, she should

    A. suction the pharynx with a catheter
    B. call the doctor
    C. both
    D. neither   (7:137)

260. In hydrocephalus, there is an excess of cerebrospinal fluid in the

    A. ventricular spaces
    B. subarachnoid spaces
    C. both
    D. neither   (7:142)

261. In hydrocephalus, there is

    A. bulging of the anterior fontanel
    B. shiny appearance of the scalp and dilatation of its veins
    C. both
    D. neither   (7:143)

262. A baby with a tuft of hair in the lumbar area should be checked carefully to rule out the existence of

    A. spina bifida
    B. dislocation of the hips
    C. both
    D. neither   (7:147)

263. Female children with adrenogenital syndrome have a

    A. small clitoris
    B. female chromosomal pattern
    C. both
    D. neither   (7:150)

264. Cardiac anomalies related to the effect of rubella virus on the fetus include

    A. septal defect
    B. patent ductus arteriosus
    C. both
    D. neither   (7:153)

265. Infants born with active syphilis often show

    A. linear scars around the mouth
    B. a persistent nasal discharge
    C. both
    D. neither   (7:155)

266. Early congenital syphilis of the infant may cause maculopapular skin rash in the

    A. back
    B. buttocks
    C. both
    D. neither   (7:155)

267. Atelectasis in the newborn is associated with

    A. distention of the aveoli
    B. cyanosis
    C. both
    D. neither   (7:161)

268. In congenital clubfoot, there is

    A. inversion of the entire foot
    B. adduction of the forefoot
    C. both
    D. neither   (7:164)

269. Early signs of congenital dislocation of the hip include

    A. increased capacity of abduction of the affected hip
    B. the gluteal skin folds being lower on the affected side

C. both
D. neither   (7:167)

270. The newborn suffers physiological weight loss during the first week of life because of

    A. loss of body fluid
    B. inadequate intake
    C. both
    D. neither   (7:171)

271. During the first year, the young infant requires daily

    A. 300 mg of vitamin C
    B. 4,000 units of vitamin D
    C. both
    D. neither   (7:178)

272. During the first year of life, the infant requires daily

    A. 50 calories/kg of body weight
    B. 10 grams of protein/kg of body weight
    C. both
    D. neither   (7:183)

273. Rich sources of vitamin D for the child include

    A. breast milk
    B. cow's milk
    C. both
    D. neither   (7:199)

274. Early clinical manifestation of scurvy include

    A. loss of appetite
    B. irritability
    C. both
    D. neither   (7:199)

275. The cause of diarrhea in an infant may be

    A. overfeeding
    B. underfeeding
    C. both
    D. neither   (7:202)

276. Vomiting in the infant may be due to

    A. swallowing too much air

B. organic obstruction
C. both
D. neither   (7:204)

277. Constipation in the formula fed baby may be the result of

    A. too little carbohydrate
    B. too little protein
    C. both
    D. neither   (7:204)

278. Obstinate constipation in the infant may be due to

    A. megacolon
    B. mechanical obstruction
    C. both
    D. neither   (7:204)

279. Vomiting in babies with pyloric stenosis causes loss of

    A. sodium
    B. hydrochloric acid
    C. both
    D. neither   (7:212)

280. Cystic fibrosis affects the

    A. heart
    B. sweat glands
    C. both
    D. neither   (7:217)

281. Cystic fibrosis affects

    A. the salivary glands
    B. the tear glands
    C. both
    D. neither   (7:217)

282. The sweat of children with cystic fibrosis of the pancreas contains low levels of

    A. potassium
    B. sodium chloride
    C. both
    D. neither   (7:219)

283. Acute bronchiolitis is

    A. caused by a viral infection

B. rarely seen before the age of 2 years
C. both
D. neither   (7:230)

284. Hemophilus influenzae pneumonia in children can cause

    A. empyema
    B. bacteremia
    C. both
    D. neither   (7:234)

285. Convulsions in children can be caused by

    A. meningitis
    B. high fever
    C. both
    D. neither   (7:236)

Each statement is followed by four suggested answers. Answer according to the following key:

    A. **if 1, 2, and 3 are correct**
    B. **if 1 and 3 are correct**
    C. **if 2 and 4 are correct**
    D. **if only 4 is correct**
    E. **if all are correct**

286. Maternal mortality includes deaths resulting from complications of

    1. pregnancy
    2. labor
    3. delivery
    4. postpartum period   (7:33)

287. Body loss of fluid in the child occurs through the

    1. lungs (breathing)
    2. skin (sweating)
    3. urine
    4. stools   (7:75)

288. Disorders associated with fluid imbalance in the child include

    1. high fever
    2. pyloric stenosis
    3. persistent vomiting
    4. severe diarrhea   (7:75)

289. Intravenous infusions for infants can be given in veins of the

   1. scalp
   2. back of the hand
   3. flexor surfaces of the wrist
   4. medial side of the ankle   (7:77)

290. Fluid therapy may consist of the administration of

   1. water
   2. electrolytes
   3. protein
   4. calories   (7:76)

291. During pregnancy, the maternal diet requires increased amounts of

   1. vitamin D
   2. riboflavin
   3. protein
   4. iron   (7:96)

292. Meconium is a sticky greenish-black substance containing

   1. bile
   2. mucus
   3. hair
   4. vernix caseosa   (7:104)

293. The newborn infant can

   1. sit up
   2. yawn
   3. whistle
   4. sneeze   (7:106)

294. In some hospitals, the umbilical cord stump of the newborn is painted daily with a triple dye containing

   1. gentian violet
   2. acriflavine
   3. brilliant green
   4. alcohol   (7:113)

295. When the infant is breast fed, there is need for a supplement of

   1. vitamin B$_{12}$
   2. vitamin K
   3. vitamin E
   4. vitamin D

296. Whether breast or bottle fed, the infant needs supplements of

   1. vitamin A
   2. vitamin B$_1$
   3. vitamin B$_6$
   4. vitamin C   (7:118)

297. The premature baby has

   1. relatively small size
   2. thick toes
   3. protruding abdomen
   4. thick fingers   (7:124)

298. The premature infant is

   1. immunologically immature
   2. prone to jaundice
   3. prone to vomiting
   4. unable to position himself   (7:126)

299. Conditions associated with the birth of premature babies include

   1. bronchial asthma
   2. multiple pregnancy
   3. cystitis
   4. placenta previa   (7:132)

300. In the noncommunicating type of congenital hydrocephalus, the site of obstruction may be at the

   1. foramen of Monro
   2. aqueduct of Silvius
   3. foramen of Lushka
   4. foramen ovale   (7:142)

Answer Key: Maternal and Child Health Nursing

1. A	39. A	77. B	115. B	153. A	191. D	229. B	267. B
2. D	40. D	78. C	116. D	154. B	192. D	230. A	268. C
3. D	41. B	79. D	117. E	155. D	193. C	231. C	269. D
4. A	42. B	80. D	118. A	156. B	194. B	232. C	270. C
5. A	43. D	81. C	119. D	157. D	195. A	233. D	271. D
6. C	44. C	82. C	120. D	158. D	196. D	234. A	272. D
7. B	45. D	83. B	121. E	159. C	197. D	235. C	273. D
8. B	46. A	84. C	122. E	160. D	198. A	236. A	274. C
9. C	47. C	85. C	123. E	161. D	199. D	237. B	275. C
10. D	48. C	86. D	124. C	162. B	200. D	238. C	276. C
11. D	49. C	87. C	125. E	163. D	201. A	239. C	277. A
12. D	50. C	88. C	126. E	164. C	202. D	240. B	278. C
13. D	51. C	89. C	127. A	165. D	203. D	241. C	279. B
14. D	52. B	90. C	128. F	166. C	204. B	242. C	280. B
15. A	53. C	91. C	129. C	167. B	205. C	243. C	281. C
16. A	54. A	92. A	130. A	168. C	206. B	244. C	282. D
17. D	55. B	93. C	131. D	169. D	207. D	245. C	283. A
18. B	56. C	94. C	132. B	170. A	208. C	246. C	284. C
19. D	57. A	95. B	133. E	171. B	209. A	247. D	285. C
20. D	58. D	96. D	134. D	172. D	210. D	248. C	286. E
21. C	59. A	97. D	135. A	173. B	211. D	249. A	287. E
22. C	60. D	98. A	136. B	174. A	212. A	250. B	288. E
23. D	61. B	99. A	137. E	175. B	213. C	251. A	289. E
24. A	62. C	100. C	138. C	176. D	214. B	252. C	290. E
25. D	63. A	101. C	139. C	177. D	215. A	253. C	291. E
26. B	64. B	102. B	140. B	178. C	216. D	254. C	292. E
27. C	65. C	103. C	141. D	179. C	217. D	255. A	293. C
28. A	66. D	104. C	142. A	180. D	218. C	256. A	294. A
29. D	67. C	105. A	143. D	181. C	219. C	257. A	295. D
30. D	68. D	106. B	144. A	182. A	220. A	258. C	296. D
31. A	69. A	107. D	145. B	183. D	221. C	259. C	297. B
32. D	70. B	108. B	146. C	184. C	222. C	260. C	298. E
33. D	71. D	109. A	147. D	185. C	223. C	261. C	299. C
34. D	72. B	110. A	148. B	186. B	224. A	262. A	300. A
35. D	73. C	111. A	149. C	187. D	225. C	263. B	
36. D	74. C	112. E	150. A	188. B	226. C	264. C	
37. B	75. C	113. D	151. C	189. A	227. C	265. C	
38. C	76. C	114. C	152. E	190. D	228. D	266. C	

Chapter Nine

Community and Public Health Nursing

Directions: Select from among the lettered choices the one that most appropriately answers the question or completes the statement.

1. A tuberculosis control program may include

    A. improved case finding
    B. treatment of active cases
    C. follow-up of persons with inactive disease
    D. all of the above   (9:493)

2. Tuberculosis is a selective disease. Case-finding techniques should be stressed in groups such as

    A. the aged
    B. pregnant women
    C. infants
    D. all of the above   (9:494)

3. Proper nutrition is related to good health. The science of nutrition includes the

    A. nutritive value of foods
    B. food requirements at different age levels
    C. food requirements in crtain diseases
    D. all of the above   (8:3)

4. The environmental source of an infection may be

    A. food
    B. water
    C. sewage
    D. all of the above   (9:272)

5. The dangerous temperatures for food at which pathogenic germs thrive are between

    A. 20 and 60°F
    B. 40 and 120°F
    C. 30 and 90°F
    D. 60 and 160°F   (8:218)

6. The most serious form of food poisoning is

    A. staphylococcal poisoning
    B. salmonellosis
    C. botulism
    D. tularemia   (8:218)

7. Foods often implicated in the transmission of salmonellosis include

    A. desiccated cocoanut
    B. cake mixes
    C. custard-filled bakery products
    D. all of the above   (8:218)

8. Rules for the prevention of food poisoning include

    A. meats should be cooked thoroughly
    B. uncooked fruits should be washed
    C. uncooked vegetables should be washed
    D. all of the above   (8:219)

9. Food-borne diseases include

    A. yellow fever
    B. tularemia
    C. poliomyelitis
    D. all of the above   (8:219)

10. All of the following diseases can be food-borne *except*

    A. septic sore throat
    B. paratyphoid fever
    C. trichinosis
    D. influenza   (8:219)

11. In certain areas, swordfish have been found to contain toxic amounts of

    A. oxalic axid
    B. mercury
    C. solanine
    D. all of the above   (8:221)

12. Food spoilage can be caused by

    A. yeasts
    B. molds
    C. bacteria
    D. all of the above   (8:227)

13. Drying is one method for preserving

    A. potatoes
    B. cereals
    C. soups
    D. all of the above   (8:228)

14. Food additives are used for all the following purposes except to

    A. increase caloric value
    B. improve flavor
    C. improve color
    D. improve nutritive value   (8:230)

15. Propionic acid can be used as a food additive in order to maintain all of the following *except*

    A. appearance
    B. alkalinity
    C. wholesomeness
    D. palatability   (8:230)

16. The functions of food additives include

    A. retention of moisture
    B. maintenance of desired consistency
    C. maturing of foods
    D. all of the above   (8:230)

17. Milk from penicillin-treated cows should be withheld from human consumption for

    A. 72 hours
    B. 48 hours
    C. 24 hours
    D. 12 hours   (8:232)

18. Community health nursing may operate under

    A. government authorities
    B. voluntary agencies
    C. health groups
    D. all of the above   (13:89)

19. The 1965 amendments to the Public Health Service Act contain provisions for extending the facilities for the care of all of the following *except*

    A. venereal diseases
    B. cancer
    C. stroke
    D. heart diseases   (13:121)

20. High-risk groups health-wise include

    A. low-income groups
    B. immature families
    C. disadvantaged families
    D. all of the above   (13:173)

21. The poor, compared to the general population, have

    A. more disability days
    B. more work days lost
    C. more hospital days
    D. all of the above   (13:212)

22. Georgia has had a viable family planning program since

    A. 1901
    B. 1912
    C. 1939
    D. 1967   (13:224)

23. In 1964, the nursing homes in the United States were serving approximately how many patients?

    A.   100,000

B. 500,000
C. 1,500,000
D. 3,000,000 (13:343)

24. In 1964, the United States had approximately how many nursing homes?

A. 2,000
B. 5,000
C. 17,000
D. 32,000 (13:343)

25. The major accrediting body for nursing homes is the

A. American Medical Association
B. American Nursing Association
C. Joint Commission on Accreditation of Hospitals
D. Department of Welfare (13:356)

26. Frequent health complaints among nursing home residents include

A. general debility
B. sensory impairment
C. dizziness
D. all of the above (13:345)

27. In confused nursing home patients, orientation can be promoted by providing

A. newspapers
B. clocks
C. calendars
D. all of the above (13:352)

28. Persons 35 to 60 years old should have a medical checkup every

A. 6 months
B. 12 months
C. 3 years
D. 5 years (13:364)

29. Booster shots for smallpox when travelling abroad are required every

A. 3 years
B. 6 years
C. 10 years
D. 15 years (13:387)

30. Protection against disease through vaccination may be needed for

A. elderly people
B. pregnant women
C. travelers
D. all of the above (13:387)

Answer the questions in this group by following the directions below. Select

A. **if only A is correct**
B. **if only B is correct**
C. **if both A and B are correct**
D. **if both A and B are incorrect**

31. Concerning food,

A. most diseases are due to faulty diet
B. starch and protein cannot be eaten together
C. both
D. neither (8:13,14)

32. Food fads and fallacies have developed from

A. nutrition education
B. food habits
C. both
D. neither (8:13)

33. Eating raw clams has been associated with outbreaks of

A. hepatitis
B. typhoid fever
C. both
D. neither (8:220)

34. Food-borne diseases include

A. measles
B. typhoid fever
C. both
D. neither (8:219)

35. Food-borne diseases include

A. malaria
B. meningitis
C. both
D. neither (8:219)

36. Stephylococcal food poisoning can be prevented by

    A. refrigerating perishable foods
    B. eliminating mosquitoes
    C. both
    D. neither   (8:218)

37. Sources of human salmonellosis include

    A. domestic animals
    B. livestock
    C. both
    D. neither   (8:218)

38. Salmonellosis can be transmitted to man from

    A. food
    B. water
    C. both
    D. neither   (8:218)

39. Foods often implicated in the transmission of salmonellosis include

    A. prepared meats
    B. bread
    C. both
    D. neither   (8:218)

40. Outbreaks of type A and B botulism can be caused by contaminated

    A. vegetables
    B. meats
    C. both
    D. neither   (8:219)

41. Outbreaks of type E botulism are usually due to contaminated

    A. milk
    B. ice cream
    C. both
    D. neither   (8:219)

42. Contaminated meat can be made safe from trichinosis by

    A. thorough cooking
    B. exposure to radioactive cobalt
    C. both
    D. neither   (8:220)

43. Certified milk

    A. has more than 20,000 bacteria/cu cm
    B. is not older than 72 hours
    C. both
    D. neither   (8:183)

44. Thorough cooking can prevent transmission of

    A. tularemia
    B. tapeworm infection
    C. both
    D. neither   (8:220)

45. Drying can be used for the preservation of

    A. bread mixes
    B. dessert mixes
    C. both
    D. neither   (8:228)

46. Drying can be used for the preservation of

    A. eggs
    B. milk
    C. both
    D. neither   (8:228)

47. Monosodium glutamate is a food additive used for improving

    A. flavor
    B. color
    C. both
    D. neither   (8:230)

48. Carotene may be used as a food additive in

    A. candy
    B. cheese
    C. both
    D. neither   (8:230)

49. Substances considered safe for use as food additives include

    A. glycerin
    B. magnesium carbonate
    C. both
    D. neither   (8:230)

50. Functions of substances used as food additives include

    A. imparting characteristic color
    B. controlling acidity or alkalinity
    C. both
    D. neither   (8:230)

51. Concerning dental health, it is important to know that

    A. fluorine in the drinking water reduces the incidence of dental caries
    B. dental caries can be completely prevented by a high protein diet
    C. both
    D. neither   (8:113)

52. A communicable disease can be transmitted to man from

    A. an infected person
    B. an infected animal
    C. both
    D. neither   (9:270)

53. The decline in the incidence of tuberculosis is due to

    A. widespread use of antituberculosis drugs
    B. increased activities of the local health departments
    C. both
    D. neither   (9:492)

54. A tuberculosis-control program may include

    A. chemotherapy for all persons with positive tuberculin test
    B. prevention of relapses in persons with inactive disease
    C. both
    D. neither   (9:493)

55. Syphilis

    A. is a reportable disease
    B. can be effectively treated with penicillin
    C. both
    D. neither   (9:477-78)

56. Concerning mental illness

    A. one person in ten in the United States suffers from some form of mental illness
    B. 55% of the hospital beds in the United States are filled with patients whose primary diagnosis is mental illness
    C. both
    D. neither   (9:118)

57. The nutritional needs of the aged

    A. do not differ much from those of young adults
    B. require large amounts of calcium
    C. both
    D. neither   (8:292,294)

58. Alcoholics Anonymous

    A. provides assistance in the rehabilitation of alcoholics
    B. is a branch of the Department of Welfare
    C. both
    D. neither   (12:263)

59. Causes of death in which preventability is high include

    A. malignant neoplasms
    B. accidents
    C. both
    D. neither   (13:10)

60. The 1965 amendments to the Social Security Act provided for

    A. prevention of infectious diseases through immunization
    B. training professional personnel in the care of crippled children
    C. both
    D. neither   (13:122)

61. The Mental Health Act of 1946 provided

    A. programs for developing health services in the various states
    B. genetic counseling for families with histories of mental disease
    C. both
    D. neither   (13:121)

62. Chronic diseases require

    A. long care

B. special rehabilitative training of the patient
C. both
D. neither   (13:121)

63. The amendments to the Social Security Act in 1965 introduced

A. Medicaid
B. Medicare
C. both
D. neither   (13:121)

64. The nurse can support a patient through the course of a chronic disease by

A. pursuing the patient's care regimen
B. maximizing the patient's comfort
C. both
D. neither   (13:125)

65. Many families need emotional support during

A. childbearing
B. early infancy
C. both
D. neither   (13:171)

66. The community nurse contributes to the reduction of maternal risk by providing

A. prepregnancy care
B. interpregnancy care
C. both
D. neither   (13:173)

67. The community nurse can help the expectant mother by helping her family to

A. provide special care that has been ordered by the physician
B. develop skills useful in childbearing
C. both
D. neither   (13:179)

68. Poor families compared to the general population show lower rates of

A. tuberculosis
B. visual impairment
C. both
D. neither   (13:212)

69. Poor families compared to the general population show lower rates of

A. cancer of the cervix
B. illegitimacy
C. both
D. neither   (13:212)

70. Poor families compared to the general population have

A. more disabling heart disease
B. less mental disorders
C. both
D. neither   (13:212)

71. The increased rate of growth of the world's population is due to

A. lack of family planning
B. advances in health care that prevent untimely deaths
C. both
D. neither   (13:223)

72. Family planning is

A. an elective health procedure
B. a preventive health procedure
C. both
D. neither   (13:224)

73. In bedridden nursing home residents there is risk of

A. decubiti
B. muscle contracture
C. both
D. neither   (13:345)

74. Frequent complaints among nursing home residents include

A. fatigue
B. hyperthermia
C. both
D. neither   (13:345)

75. Most residents of nursing homes

A. have a chronic illness requiring intensive medical care
B. are elderly

C. both
D. neither   (13:345)

76. Disorders found often in nursing home residents include

    A. glaucoma
    B. diphtheria
    C. both
    D. neither   (13:345)

77. The care required for nursing home residents is provided by

    A. professional personnel
    B. nonprofessional personnel
    C. both
    D. neither   (13:352)

78. Accreditation of nursing homes is based on

    A. number of nurses available
    B. surveys made by experts in the field
    C. both
    D. neither   (13:356)

79. A medical checkup is required every

    A. two months for persons over 60 years of age
    B. three months for babies during the first 6 months of age
    C. both
    D. neither   (13:364)

80. A medical checkup is recommended

    A. twice a year for children 2 to 5 years of age
    B. every 5 years for persons 15 to 35 years of age
    C. both
    D. neither   (13:364)

81. Protection against disease through vaccination may be needed for

    A. employees with high exposure to disease
    B. persons living in groups
    C. both
    D. neither   (13:387)

82. Home care of communicable diseases is limited to

    A. minor communicable diseases
    B. long-term illnesses that are under reasonable control
    C. both
    D. neither   (13:388)

83. The community health nurse can contribute to venereal disease case findings by

    A. contact tracing
    B. participating in screening measures
    C. both
    D. neither   (13:390)

84. Decreased resistance to tuberculosis is associated with

    A. malnutrition
    B. poor personal hygiene
    C. both
    D. neither   (13:393)

Each statement is followed by four suggested answers. Answer according to the following key:

    A. if 1, 2 and 3 are correct
    B. if 1 and 3 are correct
    C. if 2 and 4 are correct
    D. if only 4 is correct
    E. if all are correct

85. The five leading causes of death include

    1. diseases of the heart
    2. accidents
    3. malignant neoplasms
    4. vascular lesions of the central nervous system   (13:10)

86. Chronic diseases causing limitation of activity include

    1. arthritis
    2. nervous diseases
    3. heart conditions
    4. gastritis   (13:11)

87. Chronic diseases

    1. are permanent

2. leave a residual disability
3. require long supervision
4. are caused by reversible pathologic conditions   (13:121)

88. Tuberculosis control programs include

    1. determination of extent of infection in contacts
    2. follow-up of those suspected of having the disease
    3. prophylactic treatment of all persons in high risk groups
    4. vaccination of all persons with active tuberculosis   (9:493)

89. Foods frequently implicated in the transmission of salmonellosis include

    1. milk
    2. milk products
    3. eggs
    4. poultry   (8:218)

90. Food-borne diseases include

    1. mumps
    2. tuberculosis
    3. herpes
    4. brucellosis   (8:219)

91. Food-borne diseases include

    1. rubeola
    2. pertussis
    3. smallpox
    4. tapeworm infection   (8:219)

92. Trichinosis can be caused by eating

    1. uncooked pork meat
    2. raw vegetables
    3. partially cooked pork meat
    4. raw clams   (8:220)

93. To prevent trichinosis, thorough cooking is required for

    1. smoked pork
    2. cured pork
    3. pork sausages
    4. shellfish   (8:220)

94. Drying can be used for the preservation of

    1. meats
    2. fish
    3. fruits
    4. legumes   (8:228)

95. Gum arabic can be used as a food additive in

    1. ice cream
    2. beer
    3. salad dressings
    4. chocolate milk   (8:230)

96. Substances considered safe as food additives include

    1. tartaric acid
    2. lactic acid
    3. citric acid
    4. fumaric acid   (8:230)

97. Specific bacteria have been added to which of the following kinds of milk?

    1. buttermilk
    2. fortified milk
    3. fermented milk
    4. homogenized milk   (8:184)

98. Drug addiction characteristics include

    1. a tendency to increase the dose
    2. a psychological need for the effect of the drug
    3. a physical dependence on the effects of the drug
    4. limitation to the lower socio-economic group   (9:128)

99. Disorders often found in nursing home residents include

    1. stroke
    2. emphysema
    3. heart disease
    4. diphtheria   (13:345)

100. To be eligible for participation in the Medicare program, a nursing home must have

    1. adequate records
    2. a physician
    3. round-the-clock nursing service
    4. an intensive care unit   (13:356)

Answer Key: Community and Public Health Nursing

1. D	14. A	27. D	40. C	53. C	66. C	79. D	93. A
2. D	15. B	28. B	41. D	54. B	67. C	80. A	94. E
3. D	16. D	29. A	42. C	55. C	68. D	81. C	95. E
4. D	17. A	30. D	43. D	56. C	69. D	82. C	96. E
5. B	18. D	31. D	44. C	57. C	70. A	83. C	97. B
6. C	19. A	32. B	45. C	58. A	71. C	84. C	98. A
7. D	20. D	33. C	46. C	59. B	72. C	85. E	99. A
8. D	21. D	34. B	47. A	60. B	73. C	86. A	100. A
9. B	22. C	35. D	48. C	61. A	74. A	88. A	
10. D	23. B	36. A	49. C	62. C	75. B	89. E	
11. B	24. C	37. C	50. C	63. C	76. A	90. C	
12. D	25. C	38. C	51. A	64. C	77. C	91. D	
13. D	26. D	39. A	52. C	65. C	78. B	92. B	

Chapter Ten

History and Law

Directions: Select from among the lettered choices the one that most appropriately answers the question or completes the statement.

1. The growth of professional nursing has been influenced by

   A. the Crusades
   B. the Reformation
   C. the Industrial Revolution
   D. all of the above (10:3)

2. The chief Egyptian physician around 3000 B.C. was

   A. Imhotep
   B. Herodotus
   C. Hippocrates
   D. Nebuchadnezzar (10:7)

3. A main center for medical care in ancient Greece was

   A. Delphi
   B. Athens
   C. Epidaurus
   D. Sparta (10:9)

4. The Mohammedan physician Rhazes was noted for his study of

   A. anesthetics
   B. communicable diseases
   C. surgery
   D. anatomy (10:11)

5. The Order of the Visitation of Mary was established by

   A. Lambert
   B. St. Joan de Chantal
   C. James Sims
   D. William Morton (10:19)

6. The Béguines were a group of lay nurses originally organized in

   A. Paris
   B. Liège
   C. London
   D. Rome (10:19)

7. St. Bartholomew's Hospital was founded in 1123 in London by

   A. Henry VIII
   B. Morgagni
   C. Prior Rahere
   D. Simon Fitzmary (10:31)

8. The oldest hospital still existing in America is the

   A. Charity Hospital of New Orleans
   B. Hotel Dieu
   C. New York Hospital
   D. Bellevue Hospital (10:55)

9. The American branch of the Sisters of Charity was founded by

   A. Pearl McIver
   B. Julia Flikke
   C. Mother Seton
   D. Clara Barton (10:55)

10. The Massachusetts General Hospital was established in

A. 1718
B. 1781
C. 1821
D. 1921   (10:57)

11. Florence Nightingale received some nursing training at the

A. Sisters of Charity
B. Kaiserwerth's
C. Butler Hospital
D. Perkin's Institute   (10:65)

12. Florence Nightingale became famous for her nursing activities during the

A. Spanish-American War
B. Civil War
C. First World War
D. Crimean War   (10:67)

13. A pioneer of reform for the mentally ill in America was

A. Mary Crossland
B. Clara Barton
C. Dorothea Dix
D. Alma Scott   (10:85)

14. The report called *Nursing for the Future* was published in 1948 by

A. Doctor Esther Lucille Brown
B. the Red Cross
C. the Rockefeller Foundation
D. Toronto University   (10:143)

15. The concept of the nursing technician was developed by

A. Doctor Brown
B. Mary Stanley
C. Lucille Petry
D. Mildred Montag   (10:148)

16. The Children's Bureau administers

A. services for crippled children
B. child welfare services
C. maternal and child health services
D. all of the above   (10:175)

17. Public health service hospitals serve

A. seamen
B. federal employees injured at work
C. personnel of the United States Coast Guard
D. all of the above   (10(189)

18. Nurses of the United States Public Health Service may serve in

A. Africa
B. Latin America
C. the Far East
D. all of the above   (10:190)

19. The first issue of the *American Journal of Nursing* appeared in

A. 1900
B. 1912
C. 1918
D. 1944   (10:218)

20. The first manual for nurses in the United States was called

A. *New Haven Manual of Nursing*
B. *News for Nurses*
C. *Registered Nurse*
D. *Textbook of Nursing*   (10:220)

21. The National League for Nursing maintains close relationships with

A. The American Medical Association
B. The American Hospital Association
C. The Federation of Licensed Practical Nurses
D. all of the above   (10:237)

22. The National Student Nurses' Association was organized in

A. 1938
B. 1943
C. 1953
D. 1962   (10:243)

23. The American Nurses' Foundation receives support from

A. the ANA
B. individuals
C. foundations
D. all of the above   (10:249)

Answer the questions in this group by following the directions below. Select

 A. **if only A is correct**
 B. **if only B is correct**
 C. **if both A and B are correct**
 D. **if A and B are incorrect**

24. During the Civil War, nursing care for soldiers was provided by

 A. the army nurse corps
 B. religious orders
 C. both
 D. neither   (10:85)

25. Services of the American Red Cross include

 A. disaster relief
 B. blood programs
 C. both
 D. neither   (10:91)

26. Nursing programs within the American Red Cross are planned with the cooperation of the

 A. National League for Nursing
 B. United States Public Health Service
 C. both
 D. neither   (10:93)

27. The report called *Nursing for the Future,* published in 1948, suggested

 A. licensure should be abolished
 B. schools of nursing should have affiliations with universities
 C. both
 D. neither   (10:144)

28. The Bolton Act in 1943 provided for

 A. grants for postgraduate education in nursing
 B. funds for hospital expansion
 C. both
 D. neither   (10:151)

29. Nurse anesthetists are needed in

 A. civilian hospitals
 B. military hospitals
 C. both
 D. neither   (10:187)

30. Schools preparing for the practice of nurse-midwifery can be found in

 A. Kentucky
 B. New Mexico
 C. both
 D. neither   (10:189)

31. The industrial nurse deals with

 A. diagnostic situations
 B. treatment situations
 C. both
 D. neither   (10:188)

32. To become a member of the Peace Corps, a nurse must be

 A. able to speak a foreign language
 B. less than 25-years-old
 C. both
 D. neither   (10:195)

33. Official publications of the professional nursing organizations in America include

 A. Nursing Research
 B. Nursing Outlook
 C. both
 D. neither   (10:217)

34. The American Journal of Nursing Company publishes

 A. *Nursing Research*
 B. *Visiting Nurses' Quarterly*
 C. both
 D. neither   (10:219)

35. Isabel Hampton Robb wrote

 A. *Principles and Practice of Nursing*
 B. *Nursing Ethics*
 C. both
 D. neither   (10:220)

36. Publications of interest to nurses include

 A. *The Catholic Nurse*
 B. *Nursing Forum*
 C. both
 D. neither   (10:220)

37. The American Association for Nurse Anesthetists

    A. was organized in 1951
    B. has an official bimonthly publication
    C. both
    D. neither   (10:244)

38. The Association of Operating Room Nurses

    A. has 40,000 members
    B. was organized in 1927
    C. both
    D. neither   (10:244)

39. Projects funded by the American Nurses' Foundation include

    A. study of the care of dying patients
    B. privacy and the hospitalization experience
    C. both
    D. neither   (10:249)

40. The American Nurses' Foundation

    A. accredits nursing schools
    B. supports research in nursing
    C. both
    D. neither   (10:249)

41. The International Council of Nurses is a member of the

    A. International Hospital Foundation
    B. American Public Health Association
    C. both
    D. neither   (10:249)

Directions: Each group of numbered words and statements is followed by the same number of lettered words, phrases, or statements. For each numbered word or statement, choose the lettered item that is most closely related to it.

Questions 42 to 46
42. Isabel Stewart
43. Isabel Adams Hampton
44. Mary Roberts
45. Mary Nutting
46. Mary Eliza Mahoney

    A. The first professor of nursing in the world
    B. One of the founders of *The American Journal of Nursing*
    C. The first professional black nurse in the United States
    D. Editor of the *American Journal of Nursing*
    E. The first nurse to receive a master's degree from Columbia University
                                 (10:101–03,135)

Questions 47 to 50
47. Amy Hughes
48. Lillian Wald
49. Linda Richards
50. Clara Barton

    A. Proposed public health nursing as a Red Cross program
    B. Became president of the American National Red Cross
    C. First school nurse
    D. America's first "trained nurse"
                                    (10:92,96)

Directions: Select from among the lettered choices the one that most appropriately answers the question or completes the statement.

51. Licensing for registered nurses is mandatory in

    A. California
    B. Connecticut
    C. Illinois
    D. all of the above   (11:13)

52. The first United States nursing practice act was adopted in 1903 in

    A. New York
    B. Florida
    C. North Carolina
    D. none of the above   (11:15)

53. Reasons for revocation of a nursing license include

    A. aiding in a criminal abortion

B. gross negligence
C. incompetency
D. all of the above (11:17)

54. A contract to be legally enforceable must contain all of the following *except*

   A. real consent
   B. incompetent parties
   C. a valid consideration
   D. a lawful object (11:26)

55. A contract

   A. implies that one person promises something
   B. implies that two persons promise each other something
   C. must be in writing
   D. none of the above (11:27)

56. All of the following are kinds of contracts *except*

   A. formal contracts
   B. implied contracts
   C. express contracts
   D. homologous contracts (11:28)

57. There is a recent trend to outlaw discrimination on the basis of

   A. race
   B. color
   C. national origin
   D. all of the above (11:46)

58. Negligence is

   A. a crime
   B. failure to act with due care
   C. a willful act
   D. none of the above (11:48)

59. The time limit within which a person having a cause of action is required to start suit is called

   A. statute of limitations
   B. a subrogation
   C. slander
   D. none of the above (11:51)

60. *Res adjudicata* is a legal term that means

   A. common sense
   B. corporate negligence
   C. usual and customary practice
   D. none of the above (11:50)

61. The circumstances of a Good Samaritan case presume that a case is

   A. unavoidable
   B. avoidable
   C. a true emergency
   D. none of the above (11:75)

62. Good Samaritan statutes provides immunity for acts of willful misconduct

   A. usually
   B. seldom
   C. always
   D. never (11:75)

63. An incident report is designed to aid

   A. in the treatment of the patient
   B. in-service education of nurses
   C. medico-legal coverage
   D. all of the above (11:84)

64. Medico-legal cases that may require reference to the nurses' notes include

   A. insurance cases
   B. personal injury cases
   C. workmen's compensation cases
   D. all of the above (11:84)

65. Overlooked sponges in surgical cases may result in liability of

   A. the surgeon
   B. the hospital
   C. the supervising nurse
   D. all of the above (11:113)

66. Minors can be examined and treated for venereal disease without consent of their parents in

   A. Maryland
   B. Connecticut
   C. Massachusetts
   D. all of the above (11:138)

67. Nurses must report child abuse in

    A. New York
    B. Virginia
    C. Ohio
    D. all of the above   (11:143)

68. Control over donations of body organs is a function of

    A. city authorities
    B. state government
    C. federal government
    D. all of the above   (11:161)

69. Homicide can be

    A. justifiable
    B. excusable
    C. a felony
    D. all of the above   (11:175)

70. The law requires that a p.r.n. order for a narcotic drug must be rewritten every

    A. 12 hours
    B. 24 hours
    C. 48 hours
    D. 72 hours   (11:182)

71. Federal Narcotic Laws include

    A. the Marihuana Tax Act
    B. the Harrison Narcotic Law
    C. the Narcotic Drugs Import and Export Act
    D. all of the above   (11:182)

72. How many states have adopted the United States Narcotic Act?

    A. 28
    B. 32
    C. 36
    D. 42   (11:182)

73. *Res ipsa loquitur* is a legal doctrine that means

    A. a presumption that negligence exists
    B. expert testimony
    C. breach of warranty of sale
    D. the amount of time involved in a contract   (11:208)

74. Which of the following are intentional torts?

    A. libel and slander
    B. assault and battery
    C. false imprisonment
    D. all of the above   (11:216)

Answer the questions in this group by following the directions below. Select

    A. if only A is correct
    B. if only B is correct
    C. if both A and B are correct
    D. if both A and B are incorrect

75. Criminal law deals with acts against

    A. the welfare of the public
    B. the safety of the public
    C. both
    D. neither   (11:5)

76. Licensing for registered nurses is mandatory in

    A. Pennsylvania
    B. New Mexico
    C. both
    D. neither   (11:13)

77. Reasons for revocation of a nursing license include

    A. drug addiction
    B. advanced age
    C. both
    D. neither   (11:17)

78. Every contract must have an

    A. offer
    B. acceptance
    C. both
    D. neither   (11:27)

79. A contract, to be legally enforceable, must have

    A. the form required by law
    B. competent parties
    C. both
    D. neither   (11:26)

80. Persons involved in a lawsuit include

    A. the plaintiff
    B. the defendant
    C. both
    D. neither   (11:49)

81. The legal principle of *respondeat superior*

    A. makes the employee not individually liable
    B. holds the employer liable for the actions of the employee
    C. both
    D. neither   (11:61)

82. The doctrine of holding a hospital liable for the actions of a nurse is known as

    A. *respondeat superior*
    B. *caveat emptor*
    C. both
    D. neither   (11:62)

83. Good Samaritan legislation is designed to encourage

    A. volunteer first aid in emergency situations
    B. care of patients by volunteers in the hospital wards
    C. both
    D. neither   (11:75)

84. An emergency situation under the Good Samaritan statutes may arise in

    A. the emergency room of the hospital
    B. a highway
    C. both
    D. neither   (11:75)

85. Functions served by the incident report include

    A. in-service education of residents
    B. administrative supervision
    C. both
    D. neither   (11:84)

86. Medico-legal cases that may need reference to the nurses' notes include

    A. will probates
    B. criminal cases
    C. both
    D. neither   (11:84)

87. Professional liability insurance covers the nurse when the nurse is

    A. morally obliged to pay
    B. legally liable to pay
    C. both
    D. neither   (11:102)

88. Negligence of professional personnel is called

    A. malpractice
    B. abandonment
    C. both
    D. neither   (11:110)

89. The administration of the wrong dosage of medication

    A. never results in the hospital's liability
    B. may result in the nurse's liability
    C. both
    D. neither   (11:119)

90. A nurse may be held negligent for giving the wrong

    A. medication
    B. concentration of the proper medicine
    C. both
    D. neither   (11:119)

91. An emergency situation exists when

    A. the patient is in the emergency room
    B. there is an immediate threat to the life or health of the patient
    C. both
    D. neither   (11:136)

92. Formal consent for a medical procedure may not be necessary

    A. when the patient knows about the procedure and does not object
    B. in case of an emergency
    C. both
    D. neither   (11:137)

93. When a procedure is performed without the patient's consent, the

    A. hospital may be liable
    B. doctor may be liable
    C. both
    D. neither   (11:137)

94. A consent, to be valid, must be

    A. given after it has been explained to the patient the nature of the procedure and the risks involved
    B. in writing
    C. both
    D. neither   (11:137)

95. If a physician treats a minor without the parents' consent, he may be liable for

    A. assault
    B. battery
    C. both
    D. neither   (11:137)

96. Every consent to a medical procedure must be

    A. signed by the patient
    B. in writing
    C. both
    D. neither   (11:137)

97. Battery means

    A. using menacing language toward another person
    B. the unlawful beating of another person
    C. both
    D. neither   (11:136)

98. Consent for surgery must be obtained from the parents if a patient is

    A. a mature minor
    B. an emancipated minor
    C. both
    D. neither   (11:137)

99. When surgery is going to affect the sex functions of the patient, the

    A. spouse's consent is desirable
    B. patient's children must consent
    C. both
    D. neither   (11:137)

100. Organ donation statutes have been enacted in

    A. Vermont
    B. Utah
    C. both
    D. neither   (11:161)

Answer Key: History and Law

1. D	14. A	27. B	40. B	53. D	66. D	79. C	92. C
2. A	15. D	28. A	41. D	54. B	67. D	80. C	93. B
3. C	16. D	29. C	42. E	55. B	68. B	81. B	94. B
4. B	17. D	30. C	43. B	56. D	69. D	82. A	95. C
5. B	18. D	31. C	44. D	57. D	70. D	83. A	96. D
6. B	19. A	32. D	45. A	58. B	71. D	84. B	97. B
7. C	20. A	33. C	46. C	59. A	72. D	85. C	98. C
8. A	21. D	34. A	47. C	60. D	73. A	86. C	99. A
9. C	22. C	35. B	48. A	61. C	74. D	87. B	100. D
10. C	23. D	36. C	49. B	62. D	75. C	88. A	
11. B	24. B	37. B	50. B	63. D	76. C	89. B	
12. D	25. C	38. D	51. D	64. D	77. A	90. C	
13. C	26. C	39. C	52. C	55. D	78. C	91. B	